OSCEsmart

50 Medical Student OSCEs
in Orthopaedics & Rheumatology

Mr. Dominic Davenport

Executive Consulting Editor:
Dr. Sam Thenabadu

Ordering Information: Quantity sales. Special discounts are available on quantity purchases by corporations, associations, and others. For details, contact the publisher at the address above.

Orders by UK trade bookstores and wholesalers please visit www.scowenpublishing.com

Although every effort has been made to check this text, it is possible that errors have been made, readers are urged to check with the most up to date guidelines and safety regulations.

The authors and the publishers do not accept responsibility or legal liability for any errors in the text, or for the misuse of the material in this book.

Publisher's Cataloging-in-Publication data : OSCEsmart 50 medical student OSCEs in Orthopaedics & Rheumatology

ISBN-10: 0-9985267-2-X
ISBN-13: 978-0-9985267-2-0

CONTENTS

Message from the authors

Doctors of all seniorities can remember the stress of the OSCE but even more so the stress of trying to study and practice for the OSCEs. A multitude of generic undergraduate and postgraduate resources can be found on line but quality, quantity, and completeness of content can vary. The aim of the OSCESmart editorial team is to bring together specialty focused books that have identified 50 core stations encompassing the essential categories of history taking, examinations, emergency moulages, clinical skills and data interpretation with a strong theme of communications running through all the stations.

The combined experience of consultants, registrars and junior doctors to write, edit and quality check these stations, promises to deliver content that is appropriate to reach a standard we would expect of new junior doctors entering their foundation internship years and into core training. It is important to know that these stations are all newly written and based at the level of clinical competencies we would expect from these grades of doctors. Learning objectives exist for undergraduate curricula and for the foundation years, and the scenarios are based and written around these. What they are not, are scenarios that have been 'borrowed' from any medical school.

Preparation is the key to success in most things, but never more so than for the OSCEs and a candidate that hasn't practised will soon be found out. These books will allow you to practice relevant scenarios with verified checklists to learn both content and the generic approach. The format will allow you to practice in groups with one person being the candidate, one the actor and one the examiner. Each scenario finishes with three learning points. Picture these as are three core learning tips that we would want you to take away if you had only a couple of days left to the exam. These OSCE scenarios promise to be a robust revision aide for the student looking to recap and consolidate for their exams, but equally importantly prepare them for life in clinical practice.

I am immensely proud of this OSCESmart series. I have had the pleasure of working with some of the brightest and most dynamic young clinicians and educators I know, and I am sure you will find this series covering the essential clinical specialties a truly robust and invaluable companion in those stressful times of revision. I must take this opportunity to thank my colleagues for all their hard work but most of all to thank my wonderful wife Molly for her unerring love and support and my sons Reuben and Rafael for all the joy they bring me.

Despite the challenging times the health service finds itself in, being a doctor remains a huge privilege. We hope that this OSCESmart series goes some way to help you achieve the excellence you and your patients deserve.

Best of luck, Dr Sam Thenabadu

Introduction to OSCESmart 50 OSCES in Orthopaedics & Rheumatology:

Musculoskeletal problems are a very common presenting complaint in primary and secondary care. As a medical student and foundation doctor you will regularly be tasked with assessing patients with acute or chronic musculoskeletal problems, whether in clinics, theatre admissions lounge or in the Emergency . As a result it should be no surprise that musculoskeletal stations are regularly assessed in OSCE examinations.

This book will present 5 common themes of OSCE station allowing a breadth of knowledge to be gained while maintaining focus on a given task.

History and examination stations have always formed the cornerstone of musculoskeletal OSCE examinations. In this chapter we reinforce the importance of a methodical history taking and a stepwise 'look-feel-move' examination but we hope to show you how to adapt your approach by applying it to common musculoskeletal cases.

There is a separate data interpretation chapter which tests your ability to synthesise information from clinical cases and investigations such as blood tests, synovial fluid analysis and radiographs, and to formulate differential diagnoses. These are essential skills for any medical student or foundation doctor.

We have a dedicated chapter aimed at introducing you to acute musculoskeletal problems. In our experience these high intensity scenarios are rarely covered during medical school training so we aim to build your confidence in managing these situations methodically.

We have selected some important scenarios for the communication chapter. An important skill as a doctor is the ability to establish a rapport with patients, elicit their concerns and address their expectations in an appropriate manner. The selected scenarios give you the opportunity to practice these skills while also testing your knowledge of some key musculoskeletal conditions.

We introduce the concept of a global examination mark, common throughout medical student OSCEs, which is awarded if the candidate takes a concise, organised and systematic approach to the station, formulates a correct diagnosis and appropriate management plan, while maintaining excellent standards of care with the patient.

I would like to thank the Executive Consulting Editor, Dr Sam Thenabadu, not just for his hard work and dedication to producing the OSCESmart series but also for the help and advice he has given me over the years. Thank you to my co-authors Alastair, Will, Amit, Andrew and Sujith for their contribution to this book.

Dominic Davenport

About the Authors

Mr Dominic Davenport

MBBS BSc MRCS

Specialist Registrar Trauma & Orthopaedic Surgery

Dominic Davenport is a Trauma & Orthopaedic Registrar on the South East Thames rotation.

He completed his undergraduate medical training at Guy's, King's and St Thomas' Medical School in 2010 and Foundation and Core Surgery training years in Chichester and London hospitals. He has a particular interest in musculoskeletal sports injuries and is currently studying for an MSc in Sports and Exercise Medicine at the University of Bath. He is also a Research Fellow for a national sports injury service.

Medical education has always been a passion and during postgraduate training Dominic has designed and delivered several undergraduate and postgraduate teaching programmes on musculoskeletal topics, including a mini-ATLS course for medical students, knee aspiration workshops for FY, CST and CMT trainees and contributing to regional e-teaching series for core surgical topics. He has received a King's College Hospital NHS Trust award for contribution to teaching and a South Thames Foundation School Leadership award. He has published articles on orthopaedic examination techniques focused on preparation for the MRCS exam and hopes to continue delivering medical education throughout his career.

Dr Sam Thenabadu

MBBS MRCP DRCOG DCH MA Clin Ed FRCEM MSc (Paed) FHEA

Consultant Adult & Paediatric Emergency Medicine
Honorary Senior Lecturer & Associate Director of Medical Education

Sam Thenabadu graduated from King's College Medical School in 2001 and dual trained in Adult and Paediatric Emergency Medicine in London before being appointed a consultant in 2011 at the Princess Royal University Hospital. He has Masters degrees in Clinical Medical Education and Advanced Paediatrics.

He is undergraduate director of medical education at the King's College NHS Trust and the academic block lead for Emergency Medicine and Critical Care at King's College School of Medicine. At postgraduate level he has been the Pan London Health Education England lead for CT3 paediatric emergency medicine trainees since 2011. Academically he has previously written two textbooks and has published in peer review journals and given numerous oral and poster presentations at national conferences in emergency medicine, paediatrics, medical education and patient quality and safety.

He has an unashamed passion for medical education and strives to achieve excellence for himself, his colleagues and his patients, hoping to always deliver this through an enjoyable learning environment. Service delivery and educational need not be two separate entities, and he hopes that those who have had great teachers will take it upon themselves to do the same for others in the future.

Co-authors

Mr Alastair G Dick BSc MRCS MBBS
Specialist Registrar Trauma & Orthopaedic Surgery

Mr William Nash MBBS MRCS BEng
Specialist Registrar Trauma & Orthopaedic Surgery

Mr Amit S Patel MBBS BSc MRCS
Specialist Registrar Trauma & Orthopaedic Surgery

Dr Andrew Rutherford MBBS MSc MRCP
Senior Clinical Fellow in Rheumatology

Dr Sujith Subesinghe BSc (Hons) MBBS MRCP MSc (Dist.)
Specialist Registrar in Rheumatology and General Internal
Medicine

HISTORY TAKING

1.1 HISTORY TAKING: Shoulder – instability and dislocation

Candidate's Instructions:

A 40-year-old rugby player comes to orthopaedic clinic with a troublesome shoulder. He has experienced multiple episodes of dislocation always during rugby matches. Most of these episodes have been treated with reduction on the field however the most recent episode last week required sedation in the emergency department. He is concerned about ongoing feelings of instability.

Please take and a focused history and present your findings to the examiner along with a management plan.

You have 6 minutes to take the history before being asked to summarise your findings to the examiner.

Examiner's Instructions:

A 40-year-old rugby player comes to orthopaedic clinic with a troublesome shoulder. He has experienced multiple episodes of dislocation always during rugby matches. Most of these episodes have been treated with reduction on the field however the most recent episode last week required sedation in the emergency department. He is concerned about ongoing feelings of instability.

The foundation year doctor in clinic has been asked to take the initial history and then summarise their findings back to the team.

After 6 minutes stop the candidate whatever stage they are at and ask them to 'please summarize your findings and your management plan from here'.

Ask the candidate what the likely diagnosis is and what further investigations they would like to organize.

Actor's Instructions:

You are a 40-year-old rugby player attending the orthopaedic clinic with a troublesome shoulder. You have had multiple episodes of dislocation always during rugby matches. Most of these episodes have been treated with reduction on the field however the most recent episode last week required sedation in the emergency department.

Your main concern now is the ongoing feeling that the shoulder is unstable. The shoulder is dislocating with minimal force and recently you have been apprehensive to do weights or put your arms above your head for fear of dislocation. This is now affecting your work as a labourer. You have not experienced any numbness or weakness in the arm following these injuries.

You are otherwise fit and well, no previous illnesses or operations.

You are worried about the need for surgery.

1.1 HISTORY TAKING: Shoulder – instability and dislocation

Task:	Achieved	Not Achieved
Introduces him/herself		
Clarifies who they are speaking to, establishes age		
Checks occupation		
Positions themselves at appropriate distance from patient and maintains eye contact		
Uses open questions to begin the history		
Elicits history any pain shoulder joint		
Asks about episodes of dislocation, number, mechanism of injury and method of reduction		
Asks about current neurovascular symptoms		
Asks about current ability to use the shoulder		
Enquires about exacerbating factors such as weight, overhead activity or matches		
Enquires specifically about impact on daily activities and function, including employment		
Asks about previous shoulder injuries and elicits long term problem		
Asks about past medical history		
Asks about drug history and allergies		
Asks about relevant family history		
Asks about smoking, alcohol and recreational drug use		
Elicits patient's concerns		
Summarises clinical history		
Offers diagnosis and relevant differential diagnoses		
Suggests appropriate initial investigations including blood tests and XR AP and Lateral of the shoulder, and MRI scan		
Examiner's Global Mark	/5	
Actor's Global Mark	/5	
Total Station Mark	/30	

4

Learning Points

- Anterior shoulder dislocations are a relatively common presentation in the emergency department and it is important to ask questions which help establish whether there has been any neurovascular injury. The classical area of numbness over the lateral aspect of the deltoid is referred to as the 'Regimental badge' sign and occurs following dislocation due to stretch of the circumflex humeral nerves.

- It is important to ascertain the age of the patient, the mechanism of injury and whether there have been previous episodes. After a single episode of traumatic anterior shoulder dislocation there is around 50% chance of another dislocation.

- Treatment options vary and evidence is controversial. It is common practice to treat first dislocation episodes with a brief period of immobilisation in a polysling following reduction. However, some advocate further investigation with MRI scan due to the association with Bankart injuries to the labrum.

1.2 HISTORY TAKING: Knee – ACL rupture

Candidate's Instructions:

A 20-year-old footballer comes to the orthopaedic clinic complaining of painless giving away of his right knee during matches and inability to twist and turn easily. He has had multiple previous injuries to the knee and no previous sought medical help although the club physio has got him back to fitness after each injury. He is now unable to play and keen for a solution to the problems.

Please take and a focused history and present your findings to the examiner along with a management plan.

You have 6 minutes to take the history before being asked to summarise your findings to the examiner.

Examiner's Instructions:

A 20-year-old footballer comes to the orthopaedic clinic complaining of painless giving away of his right knee during matches and inability to twist and turn easily. He has had multiple previous injuries to the knee and no previous sought medical help although the club physio has got him back to fitness after each injury.

The foundation year doctor in clinic has been asked to take the initial history and then summarize their findings back to you.

After 6 minutes stop the candidate whatever stage they are at and ask them to 'please summarize your findings and your management plan from here'.

Ask the candidate what the likely diagnosis is and what further investigations they would like to organize.

Actor's Instructions:

A 20-year-old footballer comes to the orthopaedic clinic complaining of painless giving away of his right knee during matches and inability to twist and turn easily. He has had multiple previous injuries to the knee and no previous sought medical help although the club physio has got him back to fitness after each injury. This doesn't affect day to day life and you can work normally.

You are otherwise fit and well, no previous illnesses or operations. You did have a few injuries in the past to the same knee all treated with rest and rehabilitation by physio. When asked about specific injuries you recall a major twisting injury around a year ago causing you to fall to the floor. You heard an audible pop and had instant swelling in the knee. You were unable to continue playing and it took 6 weeks before returning to matches.

You are worried about the need for surgery.

1.2 HISTORY TAKING: Knee – ACL rupture

Task:	Achieved	Not Achieved
Introduces him/herself		
Clarifies who they are speaking to and establishes age		
Checks occupation		
Positions themselves at appropriate distance from patient and maintains eye contact		
Uses open questions to begin the history		
Elicits history any pain in the knee		
Asks about episodes of giving way		
Asks about swelling and stiffness after giving way		
Enquires about alleviating and exacerbating factors e.g. football vs walking		
Enquires specifically about impact on daily activities and function, including employment		
Asks about previous knee injuries		
Elicits severity of previous injury a year ago		
Asks about past medical history		
Asks about drug history and allergies		
Asks about relevant family history		
Asks about smoking, alcohol and recreational drug use		
Elicits patient's concerns		
Summarises clinical history		
Offers diagnosis and relevant differential diagnoses		
Suggests appropriate initial investigations including blood tests and XR AP and Lateral of the knee, and MRI scan		
Examiner's Global Mark	/5	
Actor's Global Mark	/5	
Total Station Mark	/30	

Learning Points

- The classical presentation of ACL rupture is the patient reporting a 'pop' in the knee during a twisting motion with the foot planted on the ground. The knee usually gives way and importantly the pain and swelling should be almost instantaneous due to a large haemarthrosis (bleeding into the joint). Other injuries such as meniscal tears or chondral injuries may not cause swelling immediately.

- It is essential to consider additional injuries when an ACL tear is identified including meniscal injury, chondral injury or the presence of another ligament injury such as MCL or PCL (multi-ligament injury).

- Don't forget that patients with ACL injury don't always attend the emergency department acutely. Some patients will present at a delayed stage complaining of instability and giving way of their knee during twisting activities when attempting to return to sport following recovery from the initial injury.

1.3 HISTORY TAKING: Hip – Osteoarthritis

Candidate's Instructions:

A 70-year-old male, retired builder has presented to orthopaedic clinics with bilateral hip and groin pain for months – now worsening in the past few weeks. He complains that he is struggling to get in and out of his car to go to the shops. Recently he has had difficulty talking his grandchildren to the park.

You are the foundation year doctor. Please take and a focused history and present your findings to the examiner along with a management plan.

You have 6 minutes to take the history before being asked to summarise your findings to the examiner.

Examiner's Instructions:

A 70-year-old male, retired builder has presented to orthopaedic clinics with bilateral hip and groin pain for months – now worsening in the past few weeks.

The foundation year doctor in clinic has been asked to take the initial history and then summarize their findings back to the team.

After 6 minutes stop the candidate whatever stage they are at and ask them to 'please summarize your findings and your management plan from here'.

Ask the candidate what the likely diagnosis is and what further investigations they would like to organize.

Actor's Instructions:

A 70-year-old male, retired builder has presented to orthopaedic clinics with bilateral hip and groin pain for months – now worsening in the past few weeks.

You have noticed the pain for a few months but in the past few weeks this has significantly worsened. When asked directly this pain has been noticed when trying to play with your young grandson. You get constant dull aching pain in both hips and groin region with no radiation down the leg. The pain can be at day or night but is worse after prolonged activity such as walking, climbing stairs and getting in and out of a car. You have no back pain, no weakness in either leg and no giving way.

You are a retired builder with a history of hypertension, T2DM and you are an ex-smoker. You have a family history of arthritis.

You are worried about the need for surgery.

1.3 HISTORY TAKING: Hip – Osteoarthritis

Task:	Achieved	Not Achieved
Introduces him/herself		
Clarifies who they are speaking to and establishes age		
Checks occupation		
Positions themselves at appropriate distance from patient and maintains eye contact		
Uses open questions to begin the history		
Elicits history of pain		
Asks about distribution		
Asks about chronology of symptoms		
Enquires about alleviating and exacerbating factors		
Enquires specifically about impact on daily activities and function, including employment		
Asks about symptoms at night		
Asks about constitutional upset (e.g. anorexia, weight loss and fevers)		
Asks about past medical history		
Asks about drug history and allergies		
Asks about relevant family history		
Asks about smoking, alcohol and recreational drug use		
Elicits patient's concerns		
Summarises clinical history		
Offers diagnosis and relevant differential diagnoses		
Suggests appropriate initial investigations including blood tests and XR AP and Lateral of the hips/ pelvis		
Examiner's Global Mark	/5	
Actor's Global Mark	/5	
Total Station Mark	/30	

1.3 HISTORY TAKING: Hip – Osteoarthritis

Learning Points

- Osteoarthritis of the hip is a common condition which has a significant impact on patient's activities of daily living and this should be reflected in your history taking. It is important to ask about independent mobility, walking aids and walking distance to understand the impact the condition has on the patient.

- Osteoarthritis of the hip may occur due to secondary causes so consider asking about developmental history, previous injuries or operations or family history of hip problems. Examples include hip dysplasia, slipped upper femoral epiphysis (SUFE) or Legg-Calve-Perthes disease.

- Non-operative treatment options include activity modification and weight loss, pharmacological agents for analgesia and physiotherapy. Most operative treatments include variations of arthroplasty (joint replacement).

Candidate's Instructions:

A 47-year old female has been referred by her GP to the orthopaedic hand clinic with a 3-month history of right hand and wrist pain which has failed to settle with activity modification and splinting.

You are the foundation year doctor. Please take and a focused history and present your findings to the examiner along with a management plan.

You have 6 minutes to take the history before being asked to summarise your findings to the examiner.

Examiner's Instructions:

A 47-year old female has been referred by her GP to the orthopaedic hand clinic with a 3-month history of right hand and wrist pain which has failed to settle with activity modification and splinting. The GP believe this could be carpal tunnel syndrome requiring surgery.

The foundation year doctor in clinic has been asked to take the initial history and then summarize their findings back to the team. The doctor should consider and directly ask about exacerbating factors.

After 6 minutes stop the candidate whatever stage they are at and ask them to 'please summarize your findings and your management plan from here'.

Ask the candidate what the likely diagnosis is and what further investigations they would like to organize.

Actor's Instructions:

You are a 47-year old female has been referred by her GP to the orthopaedic hand clinic with a 3-month history of right hand and wrist pain which has failed to settle with activity modification and splinting.

You have noticed that the pain in the hand and wrist is particularly severe overnight and can wake you at night. Other exacerbating factors include using the telephone and typing on the computer. Over the last few weeks you have noticed pins and needles and altered sensation in your thumb tip and index finger. This can occur at night and required you to 'shake' your hand before it feels normal again. These symptoms prompted use of a split from the GP but no improvement.

You have had similar symptoms 3 years ago around the time of birth of you daughter which resolved spontaneously. You have no other past medical history but a strong family history of hypothyroidism. You have no allergies. You are a current smoker but consume no alcohol. You are married and have 2 children and have completed your family.

You have had trouble in functioning at work due to pain when typing and writing and your grip feels weaker. Fortunately, your employers have been very accommodating and understanding.

You are worried about the need for surgery.

1.4 HISTORY TAKING: Hand – Carpal Tunnel Syndrome

Task:	Achieved	Not Achieved
Introduces him/herself		
Clarifies who they are speaking to and establishes age		
Checks occupation		
Positions themselves at appropriate distance from patient and maintains eye contact		
Uses open questions to begin the history		
Elicits history of pain, paresthesia and weakness		
Asks about distribution		
Asks about chronology of symptoms		
Enquires about alleviating and exacerbating factors		
Enquires specifically about impact on daily activities and function, including employment		
Asks about symptoms at night		
Asks about constitutional upset (e.g. anorexia, weight loss and fevers)		
Asks about past medical history including precipitators such as diabetes and hypothyroidism		
Asks about drug history and allergies		
Asks about relevant family history		
Asks about smoking, alcohol and recreational drug use		
Elicits patient's concerns		
Summarises clinical history		
Offers diagnosis and relevant differential diagnoses		
Suggests initial investigations including X-Ray of hands, blood tests for thyroid function, inflammatory markers and FBC, Renal and Liver profiles		
Examiner's Global Mark	/5	
Actor's Global Mark	/5	
Total Station Mark	/30	

Learning Points

- When assessing a patient with potential carpal tunnel syndrome be aware of potential risk factors associated with the condition such as female gender, pregnancy, obesity, hypothyroidism, diabetes and rheumatoid arthritis.

- When asking about pain always remember that apart from the classical distribution of pain and paraesthesia in the hand, patients may report some pain radiating into the forearm due to recurrent innervation.

- Remember with all hand cases to ask about clumsiness and ask specific probing questions about the ability to perform activities requiring fine dexterity such as doing up short buttons or picking up coins.

1.5 HISTORY TAKING: Spine – Cauda Equina Syndrome

Candidate's Instructions:

A 30-year-old female has presented to the emergency department with a sudden onset history of lumbar spine pain radiating down both legs and affecting her walking. She has reported previous lower back pain to her GP last year which resolved with Physio.

You are the foundation year doctor in the Emergency Department. Please take and a focused history and present your findings to the examiner along with a management plan.

You have 6 minutes to take the history before being asked to summarise your findings to the examiner.

Examiner's Instructions:

A 30-year-old female has self-presented to the emergency department with a sudden onset lumbar spine pain over the last few hours. The lower back pain did occur last year and resolved with physiotherapy. This time the pain is severe despite ibuprofen and radiates down both legs. You report weakness in both legs and difficulty walking. She has red flag symptoms of difficulty passing urine without any urgency to go. On further questioning, the patient will disclose a history of perianal sensory loss and difficulty passing urine over the past 4 hours.

The foundation year doctor in the emergency department has been asked to take the initial history and then summarize their findings back to the team.

After 6 minutes stop the candidate whatever stage they are at and ask them to 'please summarize your findings and your investigation and management plan from here'.

Ask the candidate what the likely diagnosis is and what further investigations they would like to organize.

Actor's Instructions:

You are a 30-year-old female has self-presented to the Emergency department with a sudden onset lumbar spine pain over the last few hours. The lower back pain did occur last year and resolved with physiotherapy. This time the pain is severe despite ibuprofen and radiates down both legs. You report weakness in both legs and difficulty walking. She has red flag symptoms of difficulty passing urine without any urgency to go. On further questioning, the patient will disclose a history of perianal sensory loss and difficulty passing urine over the past 4 hours.

You haven't passed urine over the last 4 hours and don't feel any urgency to pass urine. There are no issues to report with bowel symptoms although your perianal region feels numb when getting dressed. You will only reveal this to the candidate if asked directly. Your mobility is affected and you feel your legs are weaker and 'heavier' than previously.

You have no significant past medical history of note. You have 2 children born by SVD – no complications. You live at home with your husband. You are otherwise fit and well with no prescription medications and you have no allergies.

Your main concern relates to your difficulty to pass urine.

1.5 HISTORY TAKING: Spine – Cauda Equina Syndrome

Task:	Achieved	Not Achieved
Introduces him/herself		
Clarifies who they are speaking to and establishes age		
Checks occupation		
Positions themselves at appropriate distance from patient and maintains eye contact		
Uses open questions to begin the history		
Elicits pattern of back and specifically bilateral leg pain		
Asks about chronology of symptoms		
Asks about alleviating and exacerbating factors relating to pain		
Checks what analgesia has been trialled		
Asks about impact on daily activities and function		
Asks about change in bowel habit		
Asks about bladder dysfunction		
Asks about other red flag symptoms of back pain including unexplained weight loss, fevers, night sweats and peripheral motor/sensory deficits		
Asks about past medical history including childbirth, current drug therapy and allergies		
Asks about smoking, alcohol and recreational drug use		
Elicits patient's concerns		
Summarises clinical history		
Offers diagnosis and relevant differential diagnoses		
Suggests initial management plan including full clinical examination neurological examination and digital rectal examination for anal tone		
Suggests investigations including MRI of thoracolumbar spine. Recognises the urgency of onward surgical referral		
Examiner's Global Mark	/5	
Actor's Global Mark	/5	
Total Station Mark	/30	

24

Learning Points

- Cauda equina syndrome is a medical emergency and requires immediate attention. Red flag symptoms including severe back pain, saddle anaesthesia, bladder or bowel dysfunction need to be assessed promptly with urgent clinical assessment and imaging (ideally MRI scan) of the lumbosacral spine. Cauda equina syndrome may be due to non-malignant processes including central disc prolapse, but in the clinical vignette described, the opinion of a clinical oncologist would be appropriate.

- The management of cauda equina syndrome may include surgical decompression, high dose intravenous steroid therapy and/or radiotherapy if neoplasia is the likely cause

- Red flag signs and symptoms of back pain include:

  - Saddle anaesthesia
  - Reduced anal tone
  - Hip or knee weakness
  - Generalised neurological deficit
  - Progressive spinal deformity
  - Urinary retention or faecal incontinence
  - Non-mechanical pain
  - Thoracic pain
  - Fevers or rigors
  - General malaise

1.6 HISTORY TAKING: Hot swollen joint

Candidate's Instructions:

A 68-year-old man has attended the emergency department with a painful swollen left ankle. He currently has difficulty weight bearing. There is no history of trauma and he has been sent to the Medical Assessment Unit for review.

You are the medical foundation year doctor. Please take and a focused history and present your findings to the examiner along with a management plan.

You have 6 minutes to take the history before being asked to summarise your findings to the examiner.

Examiner's Instructions:

A 68-year-old man has attended the emergency department with a rapid onset of pain and swelling affecting the left ankle. The pain is very severe and he is unable to walk. He has multiple risk factors for gout including hypertension, diuretic use, diabetes and alcohol consumption.

After 6 minutes stop the candidate whatever stage they are at and ask them to 'please summarize your findings and your investigation and management plan from here'.

Ask the candidate what the likely diagnosis is and what further investigations they would like to organize. You would expect their top differential to be Gout.

Other possible differentials would be:

1. Septic arthritis (can be polyarticular in approximately 15% of cases and higher is the underlying pathogen is streptococcus)
2. Calcium pyrophosphate deposition disease (also known as pseudogout)
3. Haemarthrosis (would be unusual in the absence of anticoagulation or trauma)

Actor's Instructions:

You are a 68-year-old man with pain and swelling affecting the left ankle. Yesterday you were fit and well but this morning you woke up and noticed that you had severe pain and swelling in the ankle. You struggled to get around the house holding onto furniture as a crutch and eventually decided to come to the emergency department.

The pain is very intense – 10/10 severity and even resting the bedsheets on the affected area is painful. You have never had anything quite like this before. Asides from the left ankle you feel well. You do not have any fevers and haven't had any recent infections.

Approximately 3 years ago you had an episode of pain and swelling affecting the big toe that lasted 3-4 days before settling spontaneously (do not volunteer this information unless asked). You never found out what caused the pain and haven't had anything further until now.

You have a history of hypertension and diabetes that was diagnosed 3 years ago. You don't think your diabetes is too bad as you only have to take tablets for it.

You take bendroflumethiazide 2.5mg od, simvastatin 40mg at night and metformin 500mg bd. You are not allergic to any medications.

You work as a pub landlord. You drink more alcohol than you should – approximately 30-40 units per week of mostly beer. You don't smoke.

You should be able to get shifts covered for the next few days but are very concerned about how the pub will cope if you are unable to work for longer than that. You are self-employed and need to be able to work.

If you have time, you will ask the patient if any of your medications could be contributing to the problem.

1.6 HISTORY TAKING: Ho aedics & Rheumatology

1.6 HISTORY TAKING: Hot swollen joint

Task:	Achieved	Not Achieved
Introduces him/herself		
Clarifies who they are speaking to and establishes age		
Checks occupation		
Positions themselves at appropriate distance from patient and maintains eye contact		
Uses open questions to begin the history		
Elicits history of joint pain asking about possible triggers and relieving factors		
Asks about previous history of joint pain / swelling		
Enquires about systemic symptoms such as fever, rigors.		
Asks about past medical history		
Takes an appropriate drug history		
Enquires about alcohol consumption and smoking status		
Assesses the impact of the pain on the patient's life and work situation.		
Offers appropriate re-assurance that acute gout is a self-limiting condition and you would not expect a prolonged absence from work.		
Gives the patient an opportunity to ask questions		
Correctly identifies that bendroflumethiazide is a risk factor for gout		
Elicits patient's concerns		
Summarises clinical history		
Offers diagnosis and relevant differential diagnoses		
Suggests investigations appropriate investigations such as X-ray, blood tests and aspiration		
Suggests initial management		
Examiner's Global Mark	/5	
Actor's Global Mark	/5	
Total Station Mark	/30	

Learning Points

- In any new presentation of a hot, swollen joint, septic arthritis is the most important diagnosis to exclude as the mortality of this condition is between 10 and 15%.

- The incidence of septic arthritis is relatively low in the UK – approximately 8 cases per 100,000 patient years. Gout and pseudogout occur much more frequently.

- This patient has multiple risk factors for gout (diuretic usage, hypertension and alcohol excess). Other risk factors include family history of gout, obesity, renal disease and a diet that is high in either meat, seafood.

1.7 HISTORY TAKING: Reactive Arthritis

Candidate's Instructions:

A 23-year-old man has attended the emergency department with a painful swollen left knee and right ankle. There was no preceding trauma and he has been sent to the Medical Assessment Unit for review.

You are the medical foundation year doctor. Please take and a focused history and present your findings to the examiner along with a management plan.

You have 6 minutes to take the history before being asked to summarise your findings to the examiner.

Examiner's Instructions:

A 23-year-old man has attended the emergency department. Two weeks ago, he had an enteric infection with watery diarrhoea. This has completely settled but he has now developed pain and swelling affecting several joints.

After 6 minutes stop the candidate whatever stage they are at and ask them to 'please summarise the history and give their list of differentials'. To score 5/5 as their global mark they should take a clear, organised and concise history and offer up a differential list including the correct diagnosis.

You would expect their top differential to be Reactive arthritis secondary to the enteric infection.

Other possible differentials would be:

1. Septic arthritis (can be polyarticular in approximately 15% of cases and higher if the underlying pathogen is streptococcus)
2. Enteropathic arthritis due to inflammatory bowel disease (less likely as the diarrhoea has now settled)
3. Psoriatic arthritis – another cause of asymmetrical oligoarthritis but we would not normally make the diagnosis without a history of psoriasis affecting either the patient or a first degree relative.
4. Disseminated gonococcal infection – an increasingly rare entity
5. Gout – unusual in this age range without any family history or other risk factors.

OSCEs in Orthopaedics & Rheumatology

Actor's Instructions:

You are a 23-year-old man with pain and swelling affecting the left knee and the right ankle. This started approximately four days ago and came on without warning. You have also noticed pain without any associated swelling along the back of the left ankle along the Achilles tendon. The pain is very severe (9/10). You have taken paracetamol but it hasn't helped at all. The pain is so severe it is keeping you up at night.

Two weeks ago, you had a severe bout of what you think was "food poisoning". You felt sick and had watery diarrhoea up to 10 times per day. There was no blood or mucous in the stool. Things settled spontaneously over 3-4 days. You aren't aware of a particular food that triggered it but things seem to be back to normal with your bowels now.

Yesterday you noticed some urethral discharge (do not volunteer this unless asked by the doctor). This was mild and has now settled. You also had some discomfort/itchiness around the eyes but this has also settled.

You have no relevant past medical history. You may get asked about psoriasis or inflammatory bowel disease. You have heard of these conditions but as far as you know neither you nor any family members suffer from them. You do not take regular medications and have no allergies.

You have not had any unprotected sex within the last 6 months. You drink alcohol on social occasions but not more than 21 units per week. You do not smoke.

Your grandfather had arthritis in his hands but this only affected him when he was older and you are not sure what kind it was. No other family members have a history of joint problems.

You currently work as assistant to the regional manager at a local office. You have already missed several days off work with the pain and are concerned about missing further time off work. You are a keen cyclist and in 6 months are planning to cycle from London to Paris. You are concerned about the possibility of not being able to make this trip.

1.7 HISTORY TAKING: Reactive Arthritis

Task:	Achieved	Not Achieved
Introduces him/herself		
Clarifies who they are speaking to and establishes age		
Checks occupation		
Positions themselves at appropriate distance from patient and maintains eye contact		
Uses open questions to begin the history		
Checks duration of illness		
Elicits the history of preceding enteric infection		
Asks about symptoms of urethritis		
Elicits history of inflammatory eye disease		
Asks about risk factors for reactive arthritis – including sexual history		
Asks about past medical history		
Asks specifically about psoriasis		
Takes appropriate drug history asking about regular medications as well as any new medications taken for the pain		
Elicits patient's concerns about impact on work		
Addresses concerns about impact on social life – specifically his planned cycling trip		
Takes an appropriate family history asking specifically about any family history of arthritis		
Elicits patient's concerns		
Summarises clinical history		
Offers diagnosis and relevant differential diagnoses		
Suggests initial management plan		
Examiner's Global Mark	/5	
Actor's Global Mark	/5	
Total Station Mark	/30	

Learning Points

- Infections that can commonly cause a reactive arthritis include
    - Enteric Infections (campylobacter, salmonella, shigella and E. coli)
    - GU infections (Chlamydia)
    - Viral (Parvovirus and Rubella in the UK and Chikungunya in the Caribbean)

- Urethritis can be a reactive phenomenon from an enteric infection as in this case and does not always represent an underlying GU infection. Other common causes of an asymmetrical oligoarthritis include psoriatic arthritis and enteropathic arthritis.

- Enthesitis (inflammation at the site of a tendon insertion) is common with seronegative arthritides. In this case the Achilles tendonitis is almost certainly related to the reactive arthritis.

1.8 HISTORY TAKING: Hand - Rheumatoid Arthritis

Candidate's Instructions:

A 40-year old female has been referred by her GP to rheumatology clinic with a 3-month history of bilateral hand and wrist pain. She has been prescribed naproxen by her GP which hasn't settled her symptoms.

You are the foundation year doctor in the clinic. Please take and a focused history and present your findings to the examiner along with a management plan.

You have 6 minutes to take the history before being asked to summarise your findings to the examiner.

Examiner's Instructions:

A 40-year-old female has been referred by her GP to rheumatology clinic with a 3-month history of bilateral hand and wrist pain. She has been prescribed naproxen by her GP which hasn't settled her symptoms. The GP is concerned about the possibility of rheumatoid arthritis. Her symptoms are highly suggestive and include pain, swelling and stiffness in a symmetrical small joint pattern.

The foundation year doctor in clinic has been asked to take the initial history and then summarize their findings back to the team. The patient will disclose a family history of rheumatoid arthritis affecting a close relative.

After 6 minutes stop the candidate whatever stage they are at and ask them to 'please summarize your findings and your management plan from here'.

Ask the candidate what the likely diagnosis is and what further investigations they would like to organize.

Actor's Instructions:

You are a 40-year-old female who works as a secretary in a law firm. You have been experiencing increasingly painful hands and wrists over the last 3 months. Your symptoms are progressively worsening. You have noticed episodes of swelling affecting your metacarpophalangeal and proximal interphalangeal joints and your wrists feel puffy. You have experienced stiffness (but no swelling) in your elbows and shoulders bilaterally. You have had difficulty removing you're the rings on your fingers and have had to remove your wedding band. Your symptoms are worse in the morning compared to the evening and the stiffness lasts over 30 minutes on waking on a daily basis.

You have seen your GP on 3 occasions over the last 12 weeks and have tried a number of anti-inflammatory agents including ibuprofen and naproxen. Although they have 'taken the edge off' the pain, you are still troubled by your symptoms and are concerned about the possibility of rheumatoid arthritis.

You are known to have a history of hypothyroidism and are medicated with levothyroxine 125 micrograms once daily. You have no allergies. You are a current smoker but consume no alcohol. You are married and have 2 children and have completed your family.

You have experienced difficulty in functioning at work due to pain when typing and writing and your grip feels weaker. Fortunately, your employers have been very accommodating and understanding.

You want an early diagnosis as your late grandmother had rheumatoid arthritis that left her in a wheelchair with marked chronic changes affecting her hands. Your main concern is preventing irreversible joint damage that would prevent you from working.

1.8 HISTORY TAKING: Hand - Rheumatoid Arthritis

Task:	Achieved	Not Achieved
Introduces him/herself		
Clarifies who they are speaking to and establishes age		
Checks occupation		
Positions themselves at appropriate distance from patient and maintains eye contact		
Uses open questions to begin the history		
Elicits history of pain, swelling and stiffness		
Asks about distribution of joint involvement		
Asks about chronology of symptoms		
Enquires about alleviating and exacerbating factors relating to joint symptoms		
Enquires specifically about impact on daily activities and function, including employment		
Asks about symptoms to differentiate from psoriatic arthritis (e.g. pattern of joint involvement, psoriatic rash/nail disease or a 1st degree relative with psoriasis)		
Enquires about extra-articular manifestations of rheumatoid arthritis (e.g. interstitial lung disease, nodules, scleritis, Sjogren's syndrome, vasculitis)		
Asks about constitutional upset (e.g. anorexia, weight loss and fevers)		
Asks about past medical history including current drug therapy and allergies		
Asks about relevant family history, focusing of autoimmune diseases		
Asks about smoking, alcohol and recreational drug use		
Elicits patient's concerns		
Summarises clinical history		
Offers diagnosis and relevant differential diagnoses		
Suggests initial investigations including X-Ray of hands or high resolution ultrasound, blood tests for autoantibody serology, inflammatory markers and FBC, Renal and Liver profiles		
Examiner's Global Mark	/5	
Actor's Global Mark	/5	
Total Station Mark	/30	

Learning Points

Rheumatoid arthritis is diagnosed according to American College of Rheumatology 2010 diagnostic criteria. The disease classically presents as a symmetrical small joint polyarthritis. Symptoms of distal joint involvement, psoriatic skin or nail lesions, dactylitis or enthesitis would suggest a differential diagnosis of psoriatic arthritis

Early recognition of symptoms, diagnosis and instigation of effective definitive therapy is associated with favourable long term outcomes with regard to preventing disability and joint damage

Although not curable, rheumatoid arthritis can be treated with disease modifying drugs and biologic therapies which can effectively control the inflammatory component of disease and help patients to achieve disease remission, a realistic possibility with current treatment paradigms.

1.9 HISTORY TAKING: Back pain - Ankylosing Spondylitis

Candidate's Instructions:

A 25-year-old male has been referred by her GP to rheumatology clinic with a 9-month history of lower back pain. He has been using regular painkillers and sought his GP's attention due to a failure of his symptoms to resolve.

You are the foundation year doctor in the clinic. Please take and a focused history and present your findings to the examiner along with a management plan.

You have 6 minutes to take the history before being asked to summarise your findings to the examiner.

Examiner's Instructions:

A 25-year-old male has been referred by her GP to rheumatology clinic with a 9-month history of lower back pain. He has taken over-the-counter Ibuprofen 400mg TDS for over 4 weeks and was recently prescribed Co-Codamol 30/500mg QDS by his GP which hasn't settled her symptoms. The GP is concerned about the possibility of an inflammatory aetiology to his pain. His symptoms are highly suggestive of an ankylosing spondylitis and include early morning stiffness, a history of bilateral Achilles tendonitis and an episode of uveitis 3 years previously which resolved with topical steroids. He has no peripheral articular symptoms.

The foundation year doctor in the clinic has been asked to take the initial history and then summarize their findings back to the team. The patient will disclose a family history of inflammatory bowel disease and psoriasis affecting two close relatives.

After 6 minutes stop the candidate whatever stage they are at and ask them to 'please summarize your findings and your investigation and management plan from here'. Ask the candidate what the likely diagnosis is and what further investigations they would like to organize.

Actor's Instructions:

You are a 25-year-old male who works as an accountant. You have been experiencing increasing lower back pain and bilateral buttock pain over the past 9-months. Your symptoms are progressive and haven't resolved despite using regular anti-inflammatories (Ibuprofen) or compound analgesia (Co-Codamol) which was prescribed by your GP. You haven't noticed any episodes of swelling affecting your peripheral joints. You have suffered with Achilles tendonitis which you had attributed to regular running. Unfortunately, due to your symptoms you have been unable to partake in physical activity over the past 6-weeks.

You have had trouble with rising from bed in the mornings due to your pain and stiffness. Additionally, you find it difficult to wash and dress in the mornings and you have been late to work on a number of occasions over the last few weeks. You have also felt increasingly fatigued but associate this with increased stress at work. Your employers are concerned by your declining performance. Your job is desk-based and you find it difficult to maintain a comfortable position after working at your desk for over an hour.

You have seen your GP on 4 occasions over the last 12 weeks. You are troubled by your symptoms and are concerned by their failure to resolve. Your late father had "a bad back" at a young age but you are unaware of the underlying cause.

You are known to have a past history of uveitis which was treated successfully by ophthalmologists 3 years previously with no recurrence. Your sister has Crohn's disease and your brother cutaneous psoriasis. You have no allergies. You are a non-smoker and are tee-total. You are single with no partner.

Your main concern relates to your difficulty in participating in regular sport and exercise.

1.9 HISTORY TAKING: Back pain - Ankylosing Spondylitis

Task:	Achieved	Not Achieved
Introduces him/herself		
Clarifies who they are speaking to and establishes age		
Checks occupation		
Positions themselves at appropriate distance from patient and maintains eye contact		
Uses open questions to begin the history		
Elicits inflammatory pattern of lower back and buttock pain and stiffness		
Asks about chronology of symptoms		
Asks about alleviating and exacerbating factors relating to pain and stiffness		
Asks about impact on daily activities and function, including employment and recreation		
Asks about associated disease manifestations including psoriasis, inflammatory bowel disease, uveitis, Achilles tendonitis, interstitial lung disease symptoms and aortic valve disease		
Asks about peripheral arthritis, enthesitis and dactylitis		
Asks about red flag symptoms of back pain including unexplained weight loss, fevers, night sweats, neurological symptoms and bladder or bowel dysfunction		
Asks about past medical history including current drug therapy and allergies		
Asks about family history of inflammatory or autoimmune diseases		
Asks about smoking, alcohol and recreational drug use		
Elicits patient's concerns		
Summarises clinical history		
Offers diagnosis and relevant differential diagnoses		
Suggests initial investigations including MRI of spine and sacroiliac joints or Sacroiliac joint X-Ray, blood tests for inflammatory markers and FBC, Renal and Liver profiles +/- HLAB27 gene testing		
Advises a trial of an alternative anti-inflammatory medication, a physiotherapy referral and if		

sustained disease activity, consideration for escalating drug therapy to biologics		
Examiner's Global Mark	/5	
Actor's Global Mark	/5	
Total Station Mark	/30	

Learning Points

- Ankylosing spondylitis is diagnosed according to modified New York criteria. Patients must satisfy at least one clinical and radiological criteria. Clinical criteria include low back pain and stiffness for > 3 months which improves with exercise but is not relieved with rest. Other clinical diagnostic criteria include a limitation of motion of the lumbar spine in both sagittal and frontal planes or a limitation of chest expansion relative to normal values corrected for age and sex. Radiological criteria include sacroiliitis on plain film imaging > grade 2 bilaterally or grade 3-4 unilaterally. MRI of spine and sacroiliac joints can detect early inflammatory lesions including bone oedema and erosive changes
- Initial therapies for ankylosing spondylitis include non-steroidal anti-inflammatory drugs (NSAIDs) and land and water-based physiotherapy programmes. Anti-TNF drugs may be indicated if disease activity is not adequately controlled with non-steroidal anti-inflammatories.

- HLA B27 gene testing is not required to make a diagnosis of ankylosing spondylitis.

1.10 HISTORY TAKING: Back pain - malignancy

Candidate's Instructions:

A 75-year-old female has self-presented to the emergency department with a 2-month history of thoraco-lumbar spine pain. She has been using regular over-the-counter pain-killers but hasn't sought her GP's attention for her complaint.

You are the foundation year doctor in the clinic. Please take and a focused history and present your findings to the examiner along with a management plan.

You have 6 minutes to take the history before being asked to summarise your findings to the examiner.

Examiner's Instructions:

A 75-year-old female has self-presented to the emergency department with a 2-month history of thoraco-lumbar spine pain. Her pain suddenly worsened over the last 48 hours. She has taken over-the-counter Ibuprofen 200mg TDS for over 4 weeks but this hasn't helped. She hasn't seen her GP for this ailment. She has red flag symptoms including nocturnal pain, unintentional weight loss (approximately 10kg over the past 4 weeks) and poor appetite. Her symptoms are highly suggestive of an underlying malignancy. She has no peripheral articular symptoms. On further questioning, the patient will disclose a history of perianal sensory loss and difficulty passing urine over the past 24 hours. She has also had one episode of faecal incontinence earlier today. Of note, she is an ex-smoker with a 30 pack-year history and has had a chronic cough for 4 months which she hasn't sought medical attention for.

The foundation year doctor in the emergency department has been asked to take the initial history and then summarize their findings back to the team.

After 6 minutes stop the candidate whatever stage they are at and ask them to 'please summarize your findings and your investigation and management plan from here'. Ask the candidate what the likely diagnosis is and what further investigations they would like to organize.

Actor's Instructions:

You are a 75-year-old female who is retired. You have been experiencing increasing thoracic and lumbar back pain over the past 2 months. You thought this was related to simple 'wear and tear' arthritis and ignored the symptoms initially. You don't like troubling your GP and have tried to self-medicate and manage your symptoms with over-the-counter Ibuprofen, 200mg TDS but this has failed to settle your symptoms fully.

Your pain has suddenly worsened over the past 48 hours and this prompted you to attend the emergency department. You have experienced 10kg unintentional weight loss over the past 4 weeks, a loss of appetite and feel increasingly fatigued. Neither rest nor activity worsens your pain but you experience pain at night which disrupts your sleep.

You are embarrassed to disclose to an episode of faecal incontinence that you experienced prior to your attendance appointment and that it has been difficult for you to pass urine over the past 24 hours. You will only reveal this to the candidate if asked directly. You have also noted a change in sensation around the perianal region. Your mobility is affected and you feel your legs are weaker and 'heavier' than previously.

You have no significant past medical history of note. You are an ex-smoker (you gave up 10 years ago but smoked over 20 cigarettes per day for over 30 years). You have had a chronic cough for 4 months but haven't sought medical attention for this. You consume no alcohol. You live at home with your husband. You are otherwise fit and well with no prescription medications and you have no allergies.

Your main concern relates to your neurological symptoms and your recent decline in health, you have a feeling that there is a sinister cause of your symptoms.

1.10 HISTORY TAKING: Back pain - malignancy

Task:	Achieved	Not Achieved
Introduces him/herself		
Clarifies who they are speaking to and establishes age		
Checks occupation		
Positions themselves at appropriate distance from patient and maintains eye contact		
Uses open questions to begin the history		
Elicits pattern of back and specifically nocturnal symptoms		
Asks about chronology of symptoms		
Asks about alleviating and exacerbating factors relating to pain		
Asks about impact on daily activities and function		
Asks about weight loss		
Asks about change in bowel habit		
Asks about bladder dysfunction		
Asks about other red flag symptoms of back pain including fevers, night sweats and peripheral motor/sensory deficits		
Asks about past medical history including current drug therapy and allergies		
Asks about smoking, alcohol and recreational drug use		
Elicits patient's concerns		
Summarises clinical history		
Offers diagnosis and relevant differential diagnoses		
Suggests initial management plan including full clinical examination including breast exam and neurological examination and digital rectal examination for anal tone		
Suggests investigations including MRI of thoraco-lumbar spine, chest X-Ray (or CT chest, abdomen, pelvis) and haematological investigations including FBC, Liver, Renal, Bone profiles and a Myeloma screen		
Examiner's Global Mark	/5	
Actor's Global Mark	/5	
Total Station Mark	/24	

Learning Points

- Cauda equina syndrome is a medical emergency and requires immediate attention. Red flag symptoms including severe back pain, saddle anaesthesia, bladder or bowel dysfunction need to be assessed promptly with urgent clinical assessment and imaging (ideally MRI scan) of the lumbar-sacral spine. Cauda equina syndrome may be due to non-malignant processes including central disc prolapse, but in the clinical vignette described, the opinion of a clinical oncologist would be appropriate.

- The management of cauda equina syndrome may include surgical decompression, high dose intravenous steroid therapy and/or radiotherapy if neoplasia is the likely cause

- Red flag signs and symptoms of back pain include:

  - Saddle anaesthesia
  - Reduced anal tone
  - Hip or knee weakness
  - Generalised neurological deficit
  - Progressive spinal deformity
  - Urinary retention or faecal incontinence
  - Non-mechanical pain
  - Thoracic pain
  - Fevers or rigors
  - General malaise

1.11 HISTORY TAKING: A limping child

Candidate's Instructions:

A 7-year-old boy is brought to the emergency department by his concerned parents. They report that he has had a 2-day history of increasing pain in his right hip and they have noticed he appears to walk with a limp. They are concerns that this may represent a fracture.

You are the foundation year doctor in the clinic. Please take and a focused history and present your findings to the examiner along with a management plan.

You have 6 minutes to take the history before being asked to summarise your findings to the examiner.

Examiner's Instructions:

A 7-year-old boy is brought to the emergency department by his concerned parents. They report that he has had a 2-day history of increasing pain in his right hip and they have noticed he appears to walk with a limp. They are concerns that this may represent a fracture. After 6 minutes stop the candidate whatever stage they are at and ask them to 'please summarise the history and give their list of differentials'

In this scenario, the underlying diagnosis is not revealed but could be transient synovitis or septic arthritis. The candidate should ask appropriate questions to rule out other differentials such as traumatic injury, juvenile idiopathic arthritis, Perthes etc. There should be an attempt to gain family history and developmental history.

After 6 minutes stop the candidate whatever stage they are at and ask them to 'please summarize your findings and your investigation and management plan from here'. Ask the candidate what the likely diagnosis is and what further investigations they would like to organize.

The candidate should offer differentials and an investigation plan which should include blood tests, particularly WCC, ESR, CRP and an AP pelvis X-ray, and right hip lateral X-ray.

Actor's Instructions:

You are the concerned mother of a 7-year-old boy who starting complaining of pain in his right hip for the past 2-days which is getting worse. You are worried that his limp indicates an acute injury.

When asked by the candidate – the pain and limping came on spontaneously 2 days ago, appears to be affecting the right hip and groin region with some radiation to the knee. The other hip is unaffected. This is the first episode of any joint pains expressed by your son.

Only when specifically asked should you state that we had a common cold and high temperature around 5 days ago requiring a day off school. This has now resolved and there have been no further fevers. There have been no previous medical problems with your son and he was a normal delivery, no developmental problem as a baby.

1.11 HISTORY TAKING: A limping child

Task:	Achieved	Not Achieved
Introduces him/herself		
Clarifies who they are speaking to and relationship to child		
Positions themselves at appropriate distance from patient and maintains eye contact		
Uses open questions to begin the history		
Establishes that the limp is associated with pain		
Asks about the site of the pain and establishes laterality		
Asks about the chronicity of the pain		
Checks whether the pain occurs at night		
Asks whether spontaneous or traumatic		
Asks about other joints being affected including in the past		
Checks for systemic symptoms such as fever, night sweat, loss of appetite		
Asks about recent illnesses		
Asks about past medical history		
Asks about birth and developmental progress		
Asks about family history of hip problems especially siblings		
Checks when last ate and drank (showing recognition of potential septic arthritis requiring washout)		
Elicits patient's concerns		
Summarises clinical history		
Offers diagnosis and relevant differential diagnoses		
Suggests appropriate investigations including AP pelvis and lateral hip X-rays and bloods tests to include WCC, CRP and ESR		
Examiner's Global Mark	/5	
Actor's Global Mark	/5	
Total Station Mark	/30	

55

Learning Points

- This is a common scenario seen in the emergency department and the differentials diagnoses depend upon the age of the child. Please see table below for a summary of key differentials, this is not a comprehensive list but rather an aide memoir for important conditions to consider.

- Septic arthritis is an important differential diagnosis to consider in the acute setting. Management of septic arthritis often requires emergency washout of the affected joint along with antibiotics to reduce the chance of damage to the articulation cartilage.

- Transient synovitis is a self-limiting condition often seen following a recent viral infection such as URTI and can mimic septic arthritis. A classic and often quoted study identified 4 parameters known as Kocher's criteria which increase the likelihood of septic arthritis including; WCC greater than, ESR greater than, inability to weight bear, and temperature greater than 38.5 degrees.

EXAMINATION

2.1 EXAMINATION: Neonatal Hip

Candidate's Instructions:

A 2-month baby has been brought to see you as the foundation year doctor in the GP clinic for a check-up. There are no developmental concerns, no significant family history and birth was SVD with no complications.

Perform or describe on a model the process of examination of the neonatal hip screening.

Examiner's Instructions:

The candidate will perform or describe on a model the process of examination of the neonatal hip screening.

Actor's Instructions:

The candidate will perform or describe on a model the process of examination of the neonatal hip screening.

2.1 EXAMINATION: Neonatal Hip

Task:	Achieved	Not Achieved
Introduces self to the patient and gains consent for examination		
Washes hands or uses alcohol gel		
Explains the examination to the family		
Exposes patient appropriately or described appropriate exposure		
Interacts with child to gain their confidence		
Comments on pelvic obliquity or lumbar lordosis		
Observes global movement of all four limbs		
Comments upon symmetry of movement		
Comments upon any muscle wasting or limb length/ size discrepancy		
Observes specifically active hip movements		
Performs gentle passive movements of the hips both sides, flexion, abduction/ adduction, internal/ external rotation		
Performs Galeazzi test (hip flexion, observe knee height discrepancy in dislocation)		
Performs Barlow test (adduction and depression)		
Performs Ortolani test (abduction and elevation)		
Describes testing gait if an older mobile child		
Describes understanding that bilateral dislocation presents with no leg length discrepancy		
Thanks family and ensures patient is comfortable		
Summarises findings and further investigations		
Offers a diagnosis and other differential diagnoses		
Washes hands or uses alcohol gel		
Examiner's Global Mark	/5	
Actor's Global Mark	/5	
Total Station Mark	/30	

Learning Points

- Screening in UK is performed routinely as part of the newborn baby check by examination following birth but controversy exists as to whether USS should be used for screening.

- Beware pitfalls; Barlow's test negative if already dislocated, Bilateral dislocations may present with apparently normal leg lengths

- If dislocation neglected >6 months then fixed flexion deformity of the hip, limitation of abduction and contracture become the predominant clinical signs

2.2 EXAMINATION: Spine – Scoliosis

Candidate's Instructions:

A 14-year-old female patient presents to paediatric clinic asymmetry of chest wall and back picked up by school nurse.
You are the foundation year doctor in the paediatric outpatient department and have been asked to examine her back.

After 6 minutes the examiner will stop you and ask you to summarise back your findings, suggest your differential diagnoses and your initial management plan.

Examiner's Instructions:

In this case a 14-year-old girl has been shown to have mild chest wall and spine asymmetry on school screening by a nurse. She has been brought to the paediatric clinic for assessment

The foundation year doctor must examine the spine and should progress to focus on examination of a scoliosis. The candidate to allowed to ask some introductory questions but the focus of the station should be examination.

After 6 minutes stop the candidate whatever stage they are at and ask them to present their findings and suggest relevant investigations and management.

Actor's Instructions:

You are a 14-year-old girl sent to paediatric clinic following a routine screening at school demonstrating asymmetry of your chest and spine. You have had no previous injuries, no pain and no weakness or numbness in the legs. You walk normally, have a good range of movement when asked to bend and no weakness or sensation loss.

2.2 EXAMINATION: Spine – Scoliosis

Task:	Achieved	Not Achieved
Introduces self to the patient and gains consent for examination		
Washes hands or uses alcohol gel		
Explains the examination to the patient and offers a chaperone		
Exposes patient appropriately or described appropriate exposure		
Observes patient from front and behind looking for symmetry of muscle bulk, scars, scoliosis, abnormal hair tufts or evidence spina bifida		
Observes from the side of the patient looking for normal curvature specifically commenting on kyphosis or lordosis		
Palpates along bony margin of spinous processes identifying any areas of tenderness and reinforcing the signs of any abnormal curve		
Palpates paraspinal musculature for tenderness		
Asks patient to perform active cervical spine movements (flexion, extension, rotation and lateral flexion)		
Asks patient to perform active lumbar spine movements (flexion, extension, lateral flexion)		
Performs Adam's forward bending test and reassesses presence of deformity/ hump		
Ask the patient to sit down and observes from behind any change in the curvature/ correction		
Assesses thoracic spine rotation with the patient is a seated position with arms across the chest		
Asks the patient the lie on the couch		
Performs a screening test of hip movements		
Performs neurovascular screening examination of ONE leg		
Thanks patient and ensures patient is comfortable		
Summarises findings and further investigations		
Offers a diagnosis and other differential diagnoses		
Suggests management plan		
Examiner's Global Mark	/5	
Actor's Global Mark	/5	
Total Station Mark	/30	

Learning Points

- Adolescent Idiopathic Scoliosis is the most common form of scoliosis in adolescents aged 10-18 years. Significant curves >30 degrees are far more common in girls than boys

- The treatment depends upon the age of presentation, the state of skeletal maturity and the degree of the curve

- Always ensure you consider associated neuromuscular conditions when presented with scoliosis particularly when scoliosis presents before 10 years of age

2.3 EXAMINATION: Spine – Sciatica

Candidate's Instructions:

A 40-year-old female patient presents to the Emergency Department with severe lower back pain or acute onset when diving into a swimming pool. She has had back pain for 6 months and previously been seen by physiotherapists with some benefit. This acute pain presents with a central lower back pain and pain radiating down her right leg. She is able to weight bear but describes pins and needles in her right foot.

You are the foundation year doctor in the Emergency Department and have been asked to examine her back.

After 6 minutes the examiner will stop you and ask you to summarise back your findings, suggest your differential diagnoses and your initial management plan.

Examiner's Instructions:

In this case a 40-year-old female patient has attended the emergency department with acute onset back pain following a dive into a swimming pool. The central lower back pain radiates down her right leg and is affecting her sensation around the right foot.

The foundation year doctor has to examine the spine and should progress to focus on examination of the sciatic nerve. The candidate to allowed to ask some introductory questions but the focus of the station should be examination.

The station should provide a tendon hammer for reflexes and you are allowed to prompt the candidate to make us of this during the examination.

After 6 minutes stop the candidate whatever stage they are at and ask them to present their findings and suggest relevant investigations and management.

Actor's Instructions:

You are a 40-year-old female patient presenting to the emergency department with severe lower back pain of acute onset when diving into a swimming pool. You have had back pain for 6 months and previously been seen by physiotherapists with some benefit. This acute pain presents with a central lower back pain and pain radiates down your right leg. If asked the nature of the pain you should describe it as a sharp, shooting pain running down the back of the leg. You feel that there are pins and needles sensation in the right foot but you can walk and have not noticed any weakness.

The candidate will introduce themselves and explain the process of the examination. They will instruct you with actions they wish to perform which may include standing, walking and lying on the bed. Please follow the candidate's instructions You are allowed to answer their questions before the examination starts.

During the examination, you are able to walk with moderate pain. The key examination finding should be acute sharp shooting pain when your right leg is lifted straight off the bed. When sensation of the foot is being tested you can feel light touch but not as strongly as the other side. You have normal power in the foot and ankle.

2.3 EXAMINATION: Spine – Sciatica

Task:	Achieved	Not Achieved
Introduces self to the patient and gains consent for examination		
Washes hands or uses alcohol gel		
Explains the examination to the patient and offers a chaperone		
Exposes patient appropriately or described appropriate exposure		
Observes patient from front and behind looking for symmetry of muscle bulk, scars, scoliosis, abnormal hair tufts or evidence spina bifida		
Observes from the side of the patient looking for normal curvature specifically commenting on kyphosis or lordosis		
Palpates along bony margin of spinous processes identifying any areas of tenderness		
Palpates paraspinal musculature for tenderness		
Asks patient to perform active cervical spine movements (flexion, extension, rotation and lateral flexion)		
Asks patient to perform active lumbar spine movements (flexion, extension, lateral flexion)		
Performs Modified Schober's Index correctly using finger tips above and below sacral dimples/ PSIS		
Assesses thoracic spine rotation with the patient is a seated position with arms across the chest		
Performs Straight Leg Raise test on ONE leg and comments on presence of radicular pain		
Follows up SLR test with either Bragard's or Lasegue's test		
Assess ankle motor function		
Assess sensation around foot and ankle		
Assesses knee and ankle reflexes using tendon hammer appropriately		
Thanks patient and ensures patient is comfortable		
Summarises findings and further investigations		
Offers a diagnosis and other differential diagnoses		
Examiner's Global Mark	/5	
Actor's Global Mark	/5	
Total Station Mark	/30	

Learning Points

- Radicular symptoms are common and history and examination should exclude red flags for cauda equina syndrome

- The sensitivity of the SLR test is aid to be increased by Lasegue's and Bragard's modifications

- Lumbar disc degeneration and root impingement can present with variable lower limb weakness or sensory loss but bilateral symptoms are a red flag

2.4 EXAMINATION: Spine – Osteoarthritis

Candidate's Instructions:

A 60-year-old female patient presents to GP practice with chronic lower back pain affecting the central lower back and sometimes radiating to the groin. This pain is worst when trying to do the gardening. She denies any sharp shooting pain or weakness or sensory disturbance.

You are the foundation year doctor in the GP practice and have been asked to examine her back.

After 6 minutes the examiner will stop you and ask you to summarise back your findings, suggest your differential diagnoses and your initial management plan.

Examiner's Instructions:

In this case a 60-year-old female patient has attended her GP practice with chronic central lower back pain and restricted movements in the absence of neurological symptoms. She also gets intermittent groin pains.

The foundation year doctor has to examine the spine and should progress to focus on examination of spinal movements but also screen the hips for OA. The candidate to allowed to ask some introductory questions but the focus of the station should be examination.

After 6 minutes stop the candidate whatever stage they are at and ask them to present their findings and suggest relevant investigations and management.

Actor's Instructions:

You are a 60-year-old female patient presenting to your GP with chronic lower back pain. This pain has been present for many years and is progressively worsening. You have noticed some restricted movements of the lower back which compromise your ability to kneel during gardening. Over the recent months you have also had dull aching pain in the groin and are worried that your hips could have arthritis. You have no weakness or sensory disturbance in the legs.

The candidate will introduce themselves and explain the process of the examination. They will instruct you with actions they wish to perform which may include standing, walking and lying on the bed. Please follow the candidate's instructions You are allowed to answer their questions before the examination starts.

During the examination you find getting in and out of chair/ bed difficult. You are able to walk normally. When the candidate asks you to bend forward or to either side you report stiffness and restricted range of movement with some pain. You have no pain or stiffness in the neck or hips. You have no weakness of loss of sensation in the legs.

2.4 EXAMINATION: Spine – Osteoarthritis

Task:	Achieved	Not Achieved
Introduces self to the patient and gains consent for examination		
Washes hands or uses alcohol gel		
Explains the examination to the patient and offers a chaperone		
Exposes patient appropriately or described appropriate exposure		
Observes patient from front and behind looking for symmetry of muscle bulk, scars, scoliosis, abnormal hair tufts or evidence spina bifida		
Observes from the side of the patient looking for normal curvature specifically commenting on kyphosis or lordosis		
Palpates along bony margin of spinous processes identifying any areas of tenderness		
Palpates paraspinal musculature for tenderness		
Asks patient to perform active cervical spine movements (flexion, extension, rotation and lateral flexion)		
Asks patient to perform active lumbar spine movements (flexion, extension, lateral flexion) commenting on restricted movements		
Performs Modified Schober's Index correctly using finger tips above and below sacral dimples/ PSIS		
Assesses thoracic spine rotation with the patient is a seated position with arms across the chest		
Asks the patient the lie on the couch		
Performs Thomas' test for fixed flexion deformity		
Performs Straight Leg Raise test - negative		
Asks patient to perform active hip movements		
Performs passive hip movements looking for pain or restricted movements - negative		
Performs brief neurovascular exam of ONE leg to demonstrate the skill		
Summarises findings and further investigations		
Offers a diagnosis and other differential diagnoses		
Examiner's Global Mark	/5	
Actor's Global Mark	/5	
Total Station Mark	/30	

Learning Points

- Dual pathology of lumbar spine OA and hip OA is common in orthopaedic clinic and symptoms can be mixed. Examination should help determine pathology.

- Practice Modified Schober's test which is commonly examined in OSCE scenarios however we would recommend being able to describe the Schober's test

- Further examination during the spine station should always involve neurovascular examination of the legs

2.5 EXAMINATION: Spine – Ankylosing Spondylitis

Candidate's Instructions:

A patient has been referred by her GP to rheumatology clinic with a 6-month history of lower back pain. They have been prescribed naproxen by their GP which hasn't settled their symptoms.

You are the foundation year doctor in the clinic and have been asked to examine the patient's spine and then summarize your examination findings back to the team.

After 6 minutes the examiner will stop you and ask you to summarise back your findings, suggest your differential diagnoses and your initial management plan.

Examiner's Instructions:

A patient has been referred by their GP to rheumatology clinic with a 6-month history of lower back pain. Naproxen prescribed by the patient's GP hasn't settled their symptoms. The GP is concerned about the possibility of an inflammatory spondyloarthropathy.

The foundation year doctor in the clinic has been asked to take perform a clinical examination of the spine and then summarize their findings back to the team. If the candidate attempts to take a clinical history, please reiterate this is a clinical examination station and eliciting a history is not required.

After 6 minutes stop the candidate whatever stage they are at and ask them to 'please summarize your findings and your planned investigations'.

5 global score marks are awarded for a systematic and fluent examination adopting a "look, feel and move" approach to assessment with good examination technique. The correct diagnosis must also be offered to achieve a top global score. Candidates should check for patient comfort through the examination by maintaining adequate eye contact and checking that patients are not in overt discomfort.

Actor's Instructions:

You have presented to your GP with a 6-month history of lower back pain. As this is an examination station, you are not allowed to provide a clinical history for the candidate. You are however allowed to interact with the candidate if they ask if you your name and age or if you have any pain on palpation of your spine.

The candidate should seek permission to examine your joints. If you are in extreme pain, you must inform the candidate and examiner.

2.5 EXAMINATION: Spine – Ankylosing Spondylitis

Task:	Achieved	Not Achieved
Introduces self to the patient and gains consent for examination		
Washes hands or uses alcohol gel		
Explains the examination to the patient and offers a chaperone		
Exposes patient appropriately or described appropriate exposure		
Undertakes initial inspection of spine from behind the patient the back looking for surgical scars, scoliosis, muscle wasting and asymmetry		
Inspects from the side of the patient looking for normal curvature of spine (cervical lordosis, thoracic kyphosis and lumbar lordosis)		
Palpates spinous processes with firm pressure identifying any areas of tenderness		
Palpates paraspinal musculature for tenderness		
Palpates over the sacroiliac joints to elicit any pain or discomfort		
Assesses cervical spine movements (flexion, extension, rotation and lateral flexion)		
Assesses lumbar spine movements (flexion, extension, lateral flexion)		
Performs Modified Schober's Index correctly		
Assesses thoracic spine movement (the patient's pelvis must be fixed to assess this appropriately)		
Assesses straight leg raise and performs an ankle dorsiflexion if straight leg raise is less than 70 degrees on either side		
Performs a brief neurovascular examination of all 4 limbs (including distal power, peripheral reflexes and peripheral pulse check)		
Offers to perform Bath Ankylosing Spondylitis Metrology indices (BASMI) including tragus-to-wall distance, lateral lumbar flexion, maximal intermalleolar distance and cervical rotation		
Thanks patient and ensures patient is comfortable		
Summarises findings and further investigations		
Offers a diagnosis and other differential diagnoses		
Suggests initial management		

Examiner's Global Mark	/5	
Actor's Global Mark	/5	
Total Station Mark	/30	

Learning points

- Ankylosing spondylitis is an autoimmune inflammatory spinal disorder that predominantly affecting young males. If untreated, the spine can become ankylosed (fused) resulting in severely limited ranges of movement in all planes. The typical 'question mark posture' is seen in advanced ankylosing spondylitis

- Spinal metrology indices can be assessed over time and can be used to either track progress or document the severity of disease based on limitation in functional movements

- Ankylosing spondylitis usually presents with lower back pain and buttock pain. This may be due to sacroiliitis. Other causes of sacroiliitis include psoriatic, enteropathic or reactive spondyloarthropathy.

2.6 EXAMINATION: GALS Examination

Candidate's Instructions:

A patient has been referred by her GP to rheumatology with a 6-month history of lower back pain. They have been prescribed naproxen by their GP which hasn't settled their symptoms.

You are the foundation year doctor in the clinic and have been asked to examine the patient's gait, arms, legs and spine (GALS) and then summarize your examination findings back to the team.

After 6 minutes the examiner will stop you and ask you to summarise back your findings, suggest your differential diagnoses and your initial management plan.

Examiner's Instructions:

A patient has been referred by their GP rheumatology clinic with a 3-month history of muscle and joint pain. The foundation year doctor in clinic has been asked to take perform a GALS examination and then summarize their findings back to the team. If the candidate attempts to take a clinical history, please confirm this is a clinical examination station and eliciting a history is not required, aside from the three screening questions (listed below) that are routine in GALS assessment.

- Do you have any pain or stiffness in your muscles, joints or back?
- Can you dress yourself completely without any difficulty?
- Can you walk up and down the stairs without any difficulty?

After 6 minutes stop the candidate whatever stage they are at and ask them to 'please summarize your findings and your planned investigations'.

Actor's Instructions:

You have presented to your GP with a 3-month history of generalised muscle and joint pain. As this is an examination station, you are not allowed to provide a detailed clinical history for the candidate. You are allowed to interact with the candidate if they ask if you your name and age or if you experience any pain during the examination. You must however answer 3 specific questions (see below) that are part of the GALS examination.

- Do you have any pain or stiffness in your muscles, joints or back?
- Can you dress yourself completely without any difficulty?
- Can you walk up and down the stairs without any difficulty?

The candidate should seek permission to examine you. If you are in extreme pain, you must inform the candidate and examiner.

2.6 EXAMINATION: GALS Examination

Task:	Achieved	Not Achieved
Introduces self to the patient and gains consent for examination		
Washes hands or uses alcohol gel		
Explains the examination to the patient and offers a chaperone		
Exposes patient appropriately or described appropriate exposure		
Asks patient 3 appropriate screening questions eg 1) do you have any pain or stiffness in your muscles, joints or back? 2) do you struggle to dress yourself? 3) do you find climbing stairs difficult?		
Undertakes initial inspection of patient whilst standing in the anatomical position from all planes. Note should be made of muscular bulk, scoliosis, spinal curvatures, abnormal swellings or obvious joint deformity or asymmetry		
Gait: assess for smoothness, symmetry and ability to turn quickly		
Spine: assess lumbar spine flexion (placing two fingers on the lumbar spine) and asking the patient to bend forward with legs shoulder width apart and keeping knees straight		
Spine: assess lateral flexion of cervical spine		
Assess temporomandibular joint movement		
Arms: assess shoulder abduction and external rotation		
Arms: assess for swelling and deformity of wrist and hands		
Arms: assess finger grip strength		
Arms: assess fine precision pinch movements		
Arms: performs metacarpophalangeal joint squeeze		
Legs: whilst the patient is supine, examines knee flexion and internal rotation of the hip		
Legs: performs patella tap		
Legs: inspects the soles of the feet for callous formation		
Legs: performs metatarsophalangeal joint squeeze		
Summarises clinical findings concisely		

Actor's Global Mark	/5	
Examiner's Global Mark	/5	
Total Station Mark	/30	

Learning points

- The GALS assessment is a screening test for mechanical or inflammatory musculoskeletal disease. If there are abnormalities noted, a comprehensive regional musculoskeletal examination should be performed. The absence of abnormalities on GALS assessment does not exclude significant pathology.

- Knowing the correct content of the GALS assessment is key. To minimise inconvenience for the patient, after initial inspection, the gait, arms and spine can be performed whilst the patient is standing. Examination of the legs should be performed whilst the patient is supine.

- The results of the GALS assessment should be documented in a table. Assuming all facets of the assessment are normal, they should be recorded as below:

	APPEARANCE	MOVEMENT
GAIT	✓	
ARMS	✓	✓
LEGS	✓	✓
SPINE	✓	✓

2.7 EXAMINATION: Shoulder – Rotator Cuff Tear

Candidate's Instructions:

A 60-year-old male patient presents to see you in an Orthopaedic elective clinic appointment complaining of restricted range of movement in the shoulder for 6 months. He reports previous shoulder dislocations as a young rugby player which were reduced in the emergency department but no surgery required. He denies neck pain or weakness and sensory disturbance distal to the shoulder.

You are the foundation year doctor in the Orthopaedic clinic and have been asked to examine his shoulder.

After 6 minutes the examiner will stop you and ask you to summarise back your findings, suggest your differential diagnoses and your initial management plan.

Examiner's Instructions:

In this case a 60-year-old male patient has attended Orthopaedic outpatient clinic with restricted range of shoulder movement over 6 months. The patient has had previous dislocations successfully reduced in the emergency department but not required any surgery. The candidate is expected to illicit weakness in rotator cuff function and exclude frozen shoulder. The candidate is in the role of an foundation year doctor and has been asked to examine the affected shoulder.

The doctor has to examine the affected shoulder. The candidate to allowed to ask some introductory questions but the focus of the station should be examination of the shoulder. If required, prompt the candidate to examine the affected shoulder only.

After 6 minutes stop the candidate whatever stage they are at and ask them to present their findings and suggest relevant investigations and management.

Actor's Instructions:

You have come to see an Orthopaedic surgeon for an appointment about your weak and restricted shoulder movements. You had a previous episode of right shoulder dislocation while playing rugby in your 20's. Your right shoulder is weak particularly when trying the lift forward and to the side above shoulder height. Whilst there is discomfort at extreme ranges of movement pain is not a major symptom. You are able to get your hand behind your back easily and most shoulder movement are preserved.

The candidate will introduce themselves and explain the process of the examination. They will instruct you with actions they wish to perform which may include standing and sitting or lying on the bed. Please follow the candidate's instructions You are allowed to answer their questions before the examination starts.

During the examination your shoulder to not be acutely tender to palpation. You are able to do a full range of movement in the shoulder with the exception that when lifting out to the side you experience weakness through the mid-range of motion. You fail to fully abduct your arm against resistance and have some weakness to external rotation.

2.7 EXAMINATION: Shoulder – Rotator Cuff Tea

Task:	Achieved	Not Achieved
Introduces self to the patient and gains consent for examination		
Washes hands or uses alcohol gel		
Explains the examination to the patient and offers a chaperone		
Exposes patient appropriately or described appropriate exposure		
Observes patient in a standing and exposed from waist up		
Palpates for temperature of the joint using back of hand		
Palpates for tenderness in joint line systematically		
Specifically palpates SCJ, ACJ, spine of scapula		
Takes the chance to test tenderness at LHB with resisted flexion of the elbow		
Asks patient to demonstrate global compound movements (hands behind head, hands behind back) – excludes frozen shoulder		
Performs passive movements of one shoulder standing behind the patient and feeling for crepitus. Should do Flex/ Ext/ Abd/ Add/ Int/ Ext rot		
Performs ACJ Scarf test		
Performs Neer's impingement test		
Assesses rotator cuff function focusing on abduction in the mid-range of motion with and without resistance		
Assesses rotator cuff function of TM/IS with resisted external rotation		
Assesses rotator cuff function of Subscapularis with resisted external rotation		
Assesses for or describes how to assess apprehension test for instability		
States that would perform neurovascular examination of the arm		
Summarises findings and further investigations		
Offers a diagnosis and other differential diagnoses		
Examiner's Global Mark	/5	
Actor's Global Mark	/5	
Total Station Mark	/30	

Learning Points

- In older patients with restricted range of shoulder movements the two key differentials are degenerative cuff tear vs frozen shoulder. Frozen shoulder affects all planes of movement both active and passive and should be easily differentiated from RCT.

- Remember that RCT pathology can be acute tears in young athletic injury or degenerative in older patients. Supraspinatus is the most important musculotendinous unit to assess and affects abduction in mid-range of arc (deltoid initiates abduction).

- Management of RCT varies between patient depending upon pathology. Be aware that tenderness of LHB or ACJ are important to determine prior to surgery as it may warrant surgical excision/ release.

2.8 EXAMINATION: Shoulder – Subacromial Impingement

Candidate's Instructions:

A 40-year-old male patient presents to see you in an Orthopaedic elective clinic appointment complaining of shoulder pain progressing over 6 months. This pain is affecting his ability to work as a builder and is particularly difficult when lifting loads above head height.

You are the foundation year doctor in the Orthopaedic clinic and have been asked to examine his shoulder.

After 6 minutes the examiner will stop you and ask you to summarise back your findings, suggest your differential diagnoses and your initial management plan.

Examiner's Instructions:

In this case a 40-year-old male patient has attended Orthopaedic outpatient clinic for shoulder pain. The candidate is in the role of a foundation year doctor and has been asked to examine the affected shoulder.

The foundation year doctor has to examine the affected shoulder. The candidate to allowed to ask some introductory questions but the focus of the station should be examination of the shoulder. If required, prompt the candidate to examine the affected shoulder only.

After 6 minutes stop the candidate whatever stage they are at and ask them to present their findings and suggest relevant investigations and management.

Actor's Instructions:

You have come to see an Orthopaedic surgeon for an appointment about your painful left shoulder. You had a previous episode of left shoulder pain 10 years ago which resolved with physio. Your left shoulder pain is particularly exacerbated when doing overhead activity and throwing. The pain affects your work as a builder.

The candidate will introduce themselves and explain the process of the examination. They will instruct you with actions they wish to perform which may include standing and sitting or lying on the bed. Please follow the candidate's instructions You can answer their questions before the examination starts.

During the examination, your shoulder to not be acutely tender to palpation. You can do a full range of movement in the shoulder. You experience acute pain in the top of the shoulder when the examiner brings your arm out to the side and above your head. This is made worse when doing the same movement with the examiner resisting you. You otherwise have normal power in the arm.

2.8 EXAMINATION: Shoulder – Subacromial Impingement

Task:	Achieved	Not Achieved
Introduces self to the patient and gains consent for examination		
Washes hands or uses alcohol gel		
Explains the examination to the patient and offers a chaperone		
Exposes patient appropriately or described appropriate exposure		
Observes patient in a standing and exposed from waist up		
Palpates for temperature of the joint using back of hand		
Palpates for tenderness in joint line systematically		
Specifically palpates SCJ, ACJ, spine of scapula		
Takes the chance to test tenderness at LHB with resisted flexion of the elbow		
Asks patient to demonstrate global compound movements (hands behind head, hands behind back)		
Performs passive movements of one shoulder standing behind the patient and feeling for crepitus. Should do Flex/ Ext/ Abd/ Add/ Int/ Ext rot		
Performs ACJ Scarf test		
Performs Neer's impingement test		
Performs scapula winging test		
Assesses rotator cuff function (Abduction, External Rotation, Lift off test)		
Assesses for or describes how to assess apprehension test for instability		
States that would perform neurovascular examination of the arm		
Thanks patient and ensures patient is comfortable		
Summarises findings and further investigations		
Offers a diagnosis and other differential diagnoses		
Examiner's Global Mark	/5	
Actor's Global Mark	/5	
Total Station Mark	/30	

Learning Points

- Shoulder examination can be difficult if the movements required aren't thoroughly practiced in advance. Also, bear in mind that you may have to describe the rotator cuff muscles responsible for each movement

- Remember that impingement presents typically with a painful arc classically described as between 60 and 120 degrees of abduction. Ensure that during the impingement test you reach this arc. Ideally abduction should be in the plan of the scapula (10-15 degrees anterior to midline)

- Shoulder apprehension tests are used for indicating instability. Due to the potential for discomfort to the patient is it most likely that the examiner will ask you to describe how you would do this test rather than make you perform it. We suggest asking the patient to lie down for this to give optimum control

2.9 EXAMINATION: Hand – Osteoarthritis

Candidate's Instructions:

A 70-year-old female patient presents to see you in a GP clinic appointment complaining of bilateral pain around the base of the thumb and difficulty with grip movements. This pain has been a problem for a long time but worsened over 6 months.

You are the foundation year doctor in the GP practice and have been asked to examine her hand.

After 6 minutes the examiner will stop you and ask you to summarise back your findings, suggest your differential diagnoses and your initial management plan.

Examiner's Instructions:

In this case a 70-year-old female patient has attended GP appointment with base of thumb pain. The candidate is in the role of an foundation year doctor and has been asked to examine the affected hands.

The doctor has to examine the affected hands and is allowed to focus on a single hand to demonstrate this skill. The candidate to allowed to ask some introductory questions but the focus of the station should be examination of the knee. If required, prompt the candidate to examine one hand only.

After 6 minutes stop the candidate whatever stage they are at and ask them to present their findings and suggest relevant investigations and management.

Actor's Instructions:

You have come to see your GP for an appointment about your painful hands. The pain has gradually worsened but has suddenly become severe with difficulty making a grip when doing tasks around the house. The pain is a dull ache; you feel the thumb movements are weak.

The candidate will introduce themselves and explain the process of the examination. They will instruct you with actions they wish to perform. Please follow the candidate's instructions. You are allowed to answer their questions before the examination starts.

During the examination you are likely to have to present your hands on a table or pillow. The candidate will make comments about the observed signs of the hands. Further examination will require the examiner to palpate hand and wrist at which point you will describe pain on palpation around the base of the thumb. Further movements around the base of thumb are restricted and painful. You have no specific pain or tenderness during examination of your other digits.

2.9 EXAMINATION: Hand – Osteoarthritis

Task:	Achieved	Not Achieved
Introduces self to the patient and gains consent for examination		
Washes hands or uses alcohol gel		
Explains the examination to the patient and offers a chaperone		
Exposes patient appropriately or described appropriate exposure		
Undertakes initial inspection of hands both dorsal and palmar		
Observes any nodules around the elbow		
The candidate describes signs of posture, muscle wasting, scars, nodules and nail changes		
Assess temperature between hands using back of own hand		
Palpates the wrist systematically including the radial styloid, ulnar styloid and DRUJ		
Palpates the wrist systematically the MCPJs, PIPJs and DIPJs		
Palpates specifically the base of thumb		
Asks patient to perform global movements such as grip, pinch and thumb opposition		
Asks patient to perform specific active movements at MCPJs, PIPJs and DIPJs		
Performs passive movements of MCPJs, PIPJs and DIDPJs looking for pain and crepitus		
Performs CMCJ grind test		
Performs STT grind test		
Palpates radial and ulnar artery		
Assesses Median, ulnar and radial nerve		
Summarises findings and further investigations		
Offers a diagnosis and other differential diagnoses		
Examiner's Global Mark	/5	
Actor's Global Mark	/5	
Total Station Mark	/30	

Learning Points

- Osteoarthritis of the hand commonly affects the small joints at PIPJs and DIPJs so look for sign of joint swelling, deformity and nodes (Bouchard's and Heberden's). Involvement of the 1st CMCJ or even the entries STT complex presents with classical squaring of thumb base and thenar muscle wasting.

- Due to the mixed nature of symptoms in the hand it is essential to assess the neurovascular status of the hands.

- Global hand and wrist movements such as grip strength and pinch grip are useful indicators or impact of hand pathology on activities of daily living

2.10 EXAMINATION: Hand – Carpal Tunnel Syndrome

Candidate's Instructions:

A 30-year-old female patient presents to see you in an orthopaedic hand clinic appointment complaining of right hand night pain, intermittent pins and needles since giving birth 2 months ago. She denies any preceding symptoms.

You are the foundation year doctor in the clinic and have been asked to examine her hand.

After 6 minutes the examiner will stop you and ask you to summarise back your findings, suggest your differential diagnoses and your initial management plan.

Examiner's Instructions:

In this case a 30-year-old female patient has been sent to the orthopaedic hand clinic with symptoms of carpal tunnel syndrome affecting her right hand since giving birth 2 months ago. The candidate is a foundation year doctor and has been asked to examine the affected hand.

The doctor has to examine the affected hand and is allowed to focus on a single hand to demonstrate this skill. The candidate to allowed to ask some introductory questions but the focus of the station should be examination of the hand. If required, prompt the candidate to examine one hand only.

After 6 minutes stop the candidate whatever stage they are at and ask them to present their findings and suggest relevant investigations and management.

Actor's Instructions:

You have come to an orthopaedic hand surgeon about your right hand. Since giving birth 2 months ago the hand is painful at night and wakes you up and is only relieved by shaking the hand. There is intermittent episodes of pins and needles in your thumb, index and middle finger during the day. This is affecting your ability to care for your new baby.

The candidate will introduce themselves and explain the process of the examination. They will instruct you with actions they wish to perform. Please follow the candidate's instructions. You are allowed to answer their questions before the examination starts.

During the examination you are likely to have to present your hands on a table or pillow. The candidate will make comments about the observed signs of the hands. Further examination will require the examiner to palpate hand and wrist at which point you will not describe any pain to palpation. Further movements will involve a prayer position or tapping over the wrist at which point you can report pins and needles in your thumb, index and middle fingers after 30 seconds.

2.10 EXAMINATION: Hand – Carpal Tunnel Syndrome

Task:	Achieved	Not Achieved
Introduces self to the patient and gains consent for examination		
Washes hands or uses alcohol gel		
Explains the examination to the patient and offers a chaperone		
Exposes patient appropriately or described appropriate exposure		
Undertakes initial observation of hands both dorsal and palmar, in particular thenar wasting		
The candidate describes signs of posture, muscle wasting, scars, nodules and nail changes		
Assess temperature between hands using back of own hand		
Palpates the wrist systematically including the radial styloid, ulnar styloid and DRUJ		
Palpates the wrist systematically the MCPJs, PIPJs and DIPJs		
Asks patient to perform global movements such as grip, pinch		
Asks patient to perform specific active movements at MCPJs, PIPJs and DIPJs		
Performs passive movements of MCPJs, PIPJs and DIDPJs looking for pain and crepitus		
Performs Phalen's test		
Performs Tinel's test		
Palpates radial and ulnar artery		
Assesses Median nerve motor function with either flexion of radial 2 digits or thumb opposition or abduction		
Assesses Median nerve sensory function with light touch and 2-point discrimination at tip of index		
Brief assessment of Ulnar and Radial nerve function as a screening tool e.g.; wrist and finger extension, finger abduction		
Summarises findings and further investigations		
Offers a diagnosis and other differential diagnoses		
Examiner's Global Mark	/5	
Actor's Global Mark	/5	
Total Station Mark	/30	

Learning Points

- Carpal Tunnel Syndrome is common, make sure you recognise the secondary causes such as pregnancy, post-partum overuse, hypothyroidism, diabetes and renal disease etc.

- Carpal Tunnel Syndrome present with classical night pain in the hand which wakes the patient and is relieved when they shake out the hand. Patients can sometimes report forearm pain too due to recurrent nerve innervation.

- Make sure you can recall the motor and sensory innervation of the median nerve to the hand which then directs you to the key signs on examination.

2.11 EXAMINATION: Hand – Rheumatoid Arthritis

Candidate's Instructions:

A patient has been referred by her GP to rheumatology clinic with a 3-month history of bilateral hand and wrist pain. They have been prescribed naproxen by their GP which hasn't settled their symptoms.

You are the foundation year doctor in the clinic and have been asked to examine the patient's hands and wrists and then summarize your examination findings back to the team.

After 6 minutes the examiner will stop you and ask you to summarise back your findings, suggest your differential diagnoses and your initial management plan.

Examiner's Instructions:

A patient has been referred by her GP to rheumatology clinic with a 3-month history of hand and wrist pain. Naproxen prescribed by the patient's GP hasn't settled their symptoms. The GP is concerned about the possibility of inflammatory arthritis.

The foundation year doctor in the clinic has been asked to take perform a clinical examination of the hands and wrists then summarize their findings back to the team. If the candidate attempts to take a clinical history, please reiterate this is a clinical examination station and eliciting a history is not required.

After 6 minutes stop the candidate whatever stage they are at and ask them to 'please summarize your findings and your planned investigations'. Ask the candidate what the likely diagnosis is and what further investigations they would like to organize.

Candidates should check for patient comfort through the examination by maintaining adequate eye contact and checking that patients are not in overt discomfort.

Actor's Instructions:

You have presented to your GP with a 3-month history of joint pain affecting the hands and wrists. As this is an examination station, you are not allowed to provide a clinical history for the candidate. You are however allowed to interact with the candidate if they ask if you your name and age or if you have any pain on palpation of your joints. The candidate should seek permission to examine your joints. If you are in extreme pain, you must inform the candidate and examiner.

2.11 EXAMINATION: Hand – Rheumatoid Arthritis

Task:	Achieved	Not Achieved
Introduces self to the patient and gains consent for examination		
Washes hands or uses alcohol gel		
Explains the examination to the patient and offers a chaperone		
Exposes patient appropriately or described appropriate exposure		
Undertakes initial inspection of hands and wrists (both dorsal and palmar aspects) looking for swellings muscle wasting, scars, skin, nail and cuticle changes		
Inspects the elbows and extensor aspects of the forearms for nodules, gouty tophi or psoriatic skin plaques		
Assesses temperature over the wrists and hands		
Palpates the radial artery pulses bilaterally		
Palpates the distal and proximal joints bilaterally with appropriate technique, commenting on boggy or bony swelling		
Palpates the metacarpophalangeal joints bilaterally with appropriate technique, commenting on boggy or bony swelling		
Palpates the palms feeling for tendon sheath thickening		
Palpates both wrists with appropriate technique, commenting on boggy or bony swelling		
Assesses active (prayer and reverse prayer movements) and passive movements of both wrists		
Assesses movement of fingers by asking patient to extend and flex fingers, abduct/adduct fingers and assesses finger/thumb opposition		
Assess finger grip strength (grip my fingers tightly), fine dexterity (undo a button on a shirt or pick up a coin) and two finger pincer grip (thumb and index finger grip strength)		
Tests for symptoms of carpal tunnel syndrome (performs either Tinel's or Phalen's test)		

Tests Median, Radial and Ulnar nerve motor and sensory status		
Summarises findings and further investigations		
Offers a diagnosis and other differential diagnoses		
Comments on impact upon ADLs		
Examiner's Global Mark	/5	
Actor's Global Mark	/5	
Total Station Mark	/30	

Learning points

- Candidates should describe the pattern joint involvement based on the number and distribution of joints involved. Monoarthritis infers single joint arthritis, oligoarthritis up to 4 joints and polyarthritis more than 5 joints. Symmetry of joint involvement may also help differentiate rheumatoid from psoriatic arthritis.

- Candidates should recognise classical features of rheumatoid arthritis including symmetrical arthropathy with established signs including volar and ulnar deviation, Z thumbs, swan-neck or Boutonniere deformities. Psoriatic arthritis is suggested by characteristic psoriatic skin or nail changes, distal interphalangeal joint involvement and dactylitis. Osteoarthritis presents with bony nodal swellings of the proximal and interphalangeal joints.

- Surgical scars commonly visualised include carpal tunnel release surgery, joint replacement and tendon transfers. If a joint has an overlying scar with no joint movement, this suggests arthrodesis.

2.12 EXAMINATION: Hip – Osteoarthritis

Candidate's Instructions:

A 60-year-old female patient presents to see you in a GP clinic appointment complaining of left hip and groin pain which is restricting her gardening. She has been troubled by the pain for 2 years.

You are the foundation year doctor in the GP practice and have been asked to examine her hip.

After 6 minutes the examiner will stop you and ask you to summarise back your findings, suggest your differential diagnoses and your initial management plan.

Examiner's Instructions:

In this case a 60-year-old female patient has attended GP appointment for hip and groin pain affecting her over 2 years. The candidate is in the role of an foundation year doctor and has been asked to examine the affected hip.

The doctor has to examine the affected hip. The candidate to allowed to ask some introductory questions but the focus of the station should be examination of the knee. If required, prompt the candidate to examine the affected hip only.

After 6 minutes stop the candidate whatever stage they are at and ask them to present their findings and suggest relevant investigations and management.

Actor's Instructions:

You have come to see your GP for an appointment about your painful left hip. The hip pain has gradually worsened over the course of 2 years which no preceding injury. The pain is a dull ache and you feel it both in the side of the hip but also into the groin crease. You are currently unable to garden or walk more than a mile without stopping due to this pain.

The candidate will introduce themselves and explain the process of the examination. They will instruct you with actions they wish to perform which may include standing, walking and lying on the bed. Please follow the candidate's instructions You can answer their questions before the examination starts.

During the examination you are able to walk with moderate pain in the left hip but getting on and off the examination couch difficult. The left hip is not tender to touch. Your hip feels stiff and you are unable to bring your knees to your chest due to stiffness. The worst pain is when the candidate rotates the hip, particularly internal rotation.

2.12 EXAMINATION: Hip – Osteoarthritis

Task:	Achieved	Not Achieved
Introduces self to the patient and gains consent for examination		
Washes hands or uses alcohol gel		
Explains the examination to the patient and offers a chaperone		
Exposes patient appropriately or described appropriate exposure		
Inspects around bedside for aids or adaptations		
Observes patient in a standing position from 3 sides		
Asks patient to walk and observes gait		
Performs and explains Trendelenburg sign		
Asks patient to lie of the bed and completes observations		
Measures and explains true and apparent leg length discrepancy		
Palpates for temperature over hip and groin crease		
Palpated for tenderness systemically around join		
Assesses passive movements of the hip including internal and external rotation		
Performs active movements of the hip including flexion, internal, external rotation, ABduction and ADduction		
With patient in prone position checks passive hip extension		
Performs Thomas' test for fixed flexion deformity		
Performs FABER / Figure 4 test		
Performs Straight leg raise test / Lasegue's test		
Suggests neurovascular exam of lower limbs		
Offers a diagnosis and other differential diagnoses		
Examiner's Global Mark	/5	
Actor's Global Mark	/5	
Total Station Mark	/30	

Learning Points

- The Trendelenburg sign is said to be positive if, when standing on one leg, the pelvis drops on the side opposite to the stance leg to reduce the load by decreasing the lever arm. By reducing the lever arm, this decreases the workload on the hip abductors. The muscle weakness is present on the side of the stance leg. A positive Trendelenburg sign could indicate abductor weakness from disuse secondary to osteoarthritis but is also present in neuromuscular weakness.

- Ensure you know the landmarks for True and Apparent leg length measurements and make sure you know how to interpret the results.

- FABER or Figure 4 tests and Straight leg raises tests are looking for differential diagnoses for the hip pain such as Ankylosing Spondylitis or Sciatic nerve impingement respectively.

2.13 EXAMINATION: Knee – Meniscal tear

Candidate's Instructions:

A 30-year-old female patient presents to see you in a GP clinic appointment complaining of knee pain and locking following a twisting injury during football.

You are the foundation year doctor in the GP practice and have been asked to examine her knee then summarize your examination findings back to the team.

After 6 minutes the examiner will stop you and ask you to summarise back your findings, suggest your differential diagnoses and your initial management plan.

Examiner's Instructions:

In this case a 30-year-old female patient has attended GP appointment for knee pain and locking following a sports injury. The candidate is in the role of an foundation year doctor and has been asked to examine the affected knee.

The doctor has to examine the affected knee. The candidate to allowed to ask some introductory questions but the focus of the station should be examination of the knee. If required, prompt the candidate to examine the affected knee only.

After 6 minutes stop the candidate whatever stage they are at and ask them to present their findings and suggest relevant investigations and management.

Actor's Instructions:

You have come to see your GP for an appointment about your painful left knee. You injured your knee playing football 4 weeks ago. At the time you remember a twisting injury, and sudden pain and swelling but you were able to continue walking. Since then the knee is painful over the lateral (outer half) of the knee and occasionally locks in one position.

The candidate will introduce themselves and explain the process of the examination. They will instruct you with actions they wish to perform which may include standing, walking and lying on the bed. Please follow the candidate's instructions You are allowed to answer their questions before the examination starts.

During the examination you are able to walk but get pain in the outer half of the knee when turning. The left knee is tender to touch in the lateral (outer half) of the knee but not elsewhere. Your knee is not stiff and has a normal range of movement but when twisting tests are done you feel acute pain.

2.13 EXAMINATION: Knee – Meniscal tear

Task:	Achieved	Not Achieved
Introduces self to the patient and gains consent for examination		
Washes hands or uses alcohol gel		
Explains the examination to the patient and offers a chaperone		
Exposes patient appropriately		
Inspects around bedside for aids or adaptations		
Observes patient in a standing position from 3 sides - anterior, side, posterior		
Asks patient to walk and observes gait		
Palpates for temperature using back of hand		
Palpates the quadriceps tendon		
Palpates for tenderness in joint line systematically		
Palpates for masses in the popliteal fossa eg Baker's cyst		
Assesses for a joint effusion; 'tap' or 'milk'		
Performs active then passive movements of the knee - flexion & extension		
Checks for posterior sag (PCL)		
Examines ACL using anterior draw or Lachmann's		
Examines MCL and LCL		
Performs MacMurray's meniscal tests		
Assesses for patella apprehension		
Summarises findings and further investigations		
Offers a diagnosis and other differential diagnoses		
Examiner's Global Mark	/5	
Actor's Global Mark	/5	
Total Station Mark	/30	

Learning Points

- Demographics and mechanism of injury are key deciding whether a patient is likely to have a sport knee injury such as meniscal tear or ACL injury compared to degenerative disease.

- Remember that symptoms and signs can fluctuate so even though patients may experience 'locking' of the knee this may not occur during the examination.

- McMurray's meniscal tests are the classical exacerbation test to assist in the diagnosis of a meniscal tear. Remember that internal rotation affects the lateral meniscus, and external rotation the medial meniscus.

2.14 EXAMINATION: Knee – Osteoarthritis

Candidate's Instructions:

A 75-year-old male patient presents to see you in a routine GP clinic appointment complaining of long term knee pain and stiffness.

You are the foundation year doctor in the GP practice and have been asked to examine his knee then summarize your examination findings back to the examiner.

After 6 minutes the examiner will stop you and ask you to summarise back your findings, suggest your differential diagnoses and your initial management plan.

Examiner's Instructions:

In this case a 75-year-old male patient has attended routine GP appointment for long term worsening knee pain and swelling. The candidate is in the role of an foundation year doctor and has been asked to examine the affected knee.

The doctor has to examine the affected knee. The candidate to allowed to ask some introductory questions but the focus of the station should be examination of the knee. If required, prompt the candidate to examine the affected knee only.

After 6 minutes stop the candidate whatever stage they are at and ask them to present their findings and suggest relevant investigations and management.

Actor's Instructions:

You have come to see your GP for a routine appointment about your painful and stiff right knee. This knee pain has been affecting you for 3 years but worsened over the last 6 months following a long walking holiday in the summer. The pain is worst during weight bearing activity and could be described as an aching pain around the front of the knee.

The candidate will introduce themselves and explain the process of the examination. They will instruct you with actions they wish to perform which may include standing, walking and lying on the bed. Please follow the candidate's instructions You can answer their questions before the examination starts.

During the examination you feel pain and stiffness in the right knee when walking or during any movement of the knee on the examination couch. You can't bend the right knee as far as the left knee. Your knee is mildly tender when palpated.

2.14 EXAMINATION: Knee – Osteoarthritis

Task:	Achieved	Not Achieved
Introduces self to the patient and gains consent for examination		
Washes hands or uses alcohol gel		
Explains the examination to the patient and offers a chaperone		
Exposes patient appropriately or described appropriate exposure		
Inspects around bedside for aids or adaptations		
Asks patient to walk and observes gait		
Observes patient in a standing position from 3 sides		
Palpates for temperature using back of hand		
Palpates the quadriceps tendon		
Palpates for tenderness in joint line systematically		
Palpates for masses in the popliteal fossa eg Baker's cyst		
Assesses for a joint effusion; 'tap' or 'milk'		
Performs active then passive movements of the knee		
Checks of posterior sag (PCL)		
Examines ACL using anterior draw or Lachmann's		
Examines MCL and LCL		
Performs MacMurray's meniscal tests		
Assesses for patella apprehension		
Summarises findings and further investigations		
Offers a diagnosis and other differential diagnoses		
Examiner's Global Mark	/5	
Actor's Global Mark	/5	
Total Station Mark	/30	

Learning Points

- Be prepared for gait assessment at the start or any lower limb examination and look around for walking aids or orthotics.

- Ensure the special tests such as Lachmann's and McMurray's meniscal tests have been thoroughly practiced to a level where you are efficient during the station.

- Active movements give you a chance to observe the likely range of movement of the affected joint before attempting passive movements. Observe carefully to avoid excessive pain during passive movement tests.

2.15 EXAMINATION: Foot & Ankle – Hallux Valgus

Candidate's Instructions:

A 70-year-old female patient presents to see you in a GP clinic appointment complaining of bilateral pain around the big toe and difficulty with some footwear. This pain has been a problem for a long time but worsened over 6 months.

You are the foundation year doctor in the GP practice and have been asked to examine her hand then summarize your examination findings back to the examiner.

After 6 minutes the examiner will stop you and ask you to summarise back your findings, suggest your differential diagnoses and your initial management plan.

Examiner's Instructions:

A 70-year-old female patient presents to see you in a GP clinic appointment complaining of bilateral pain around the big toe and difficulty with some footwear. This pain has been a problem for a long time but worsened over 6 months.

The foundation year doctor has to examine the affected feet and is allowed to focus on a single foot to demonstrate this skill. The candidate to allowed to ask some introductory questions but the focus of the station should be examination of the foot. If required, prompt the candidate to examine one hand only.

After 6 minutes stop the candidate whatever stage they are at and ask them to present their findings and suggest relevant investigations and management.

Actor's Instructions:

A 70-year-old female patient presents to see you in a GP clinic appointment complaining of bilateral pain around the big toe and difficulty with some footwear. This pain has been a problem for a long time but worsened over 6 months.

The candidate will introduce themselves and explain the process of the examination. They will instruct you with actions they wish to perform. Please follow the candidate's instructions. You can answer their questions before the examination starts.

During the examination you are likely to have to present your feet. The candidate will make comments about the observed signs of the feet. Further examination will require the examiner to palpate foot and ankle at which point you will describe pain on palpation around the big toes affecting the joints. You have no specific pain or tenderness during examination of your other digits.

2.15 EXAMINATION: Foot & Ankle – Hallux Valgus

Task:	Achieved	Not Achieved
Introduces self to the patient and gains consent for examination		
Washes hands or uses alcohol gel		
Explains the examination to the patient and offers a chaperone		
Exposes patient appropriately or described appropriate exposure		
Undertakes initial observation of both feet while weight bearing from front, side and behind		
Observes medial arch and position of calcaneus in standing and tip toe position		
Asks patient to walk and observes gait		
The candidate describes signs of posture, muscle wasting, scars, nodules and nail changes		
Assess temperature between feet using back of own hand		
Palpates the foot and ankle systematically from forefoot, midfoot, hindfoot		
Palpates the ankle joint circumferentially including medial and lateral malleoli		
Palpates specifically the 1st MTPJ		
Asks patient to perform specific active movements of dorsiflexion, plantarflexion, inversion and eversion at the ankle		
Performs passive movements of IPJs, MTPJs		
Performs passive movement of midfoot, hindfoot		
Performs passive ankle movements		
Palpates dorsalis pedis and posterior tibial pulses		
Assesses distal neurology including sole of foot		
Summarises findings and further investigations		
Offers a diagnosis and other differential diagnoses		
Examiner's Global Mark	/5	
Actor's Global Mark	/5	
Total Station Mark	/30	

Learning Points

- Hallux Valgus is a complex deformity of the first digit. The condition is associated with lesser toe deformity such as 'hammer toe' and callosities on the pressure points

- Examination of the foot and ankle is daunting and infrequently practised in isolation. It is important to remember that there are multiple joints to assess for passive and active ranges of movement. The tibio-talar joint, subtalar joint and midtarsal joints should each be tested independently

- Compared to other examination stations observation and gait during assessment of the foot and ankle provide a greater proportion of the information needed to form a differential diagnosis. Ensure that you can describe the appearance of common foot and ankle pathologies.

2.16 EXAMINATION: Upper Limb Neurology

Candidate's Instructions:

A 40-year-old female patient presents to the emergency department with severe neck pain of acute onset after a low energy collision as the driver of a car. Her neck pain is constant, severe and radiates down her right arm. On and off she reports tingling sensation in the arm.

You are the foundation year doctor in the emergency department and have been asked to perform a neurological examination of her upper limbs then summarize your examination findings back to the examiner.

After 6 minutes the examiner will stop you and ask you to summarise back your findings, suggest your differential diagnoses and your initial management plan.

Examiner's Instructions:

A 40-year-old female patient presents to the emergency department with severe neck pain of acute onset after a low energy collision as the driver of a car. Her neck pain is constant, severe and radiates down her right arm. On and off she reports tingling sensation in the arm.

The foundation year doctor has to examine the upper limb neurological status. The candidate to allowed to ask some introductory questions but the focus of the station should be examination.

The station should provide a tendon hammer for reflexes and you are allowed to prompt the candidate to make us of this during the examination.

After 6 minutes stop the candidate whatever stage they are at and ask them to present their findings and suggest relevant investigations and management.

Actor's Instructions:

You are a 40-year-old female patient presents to the emergency department with severe neck pain of acute onset after a low energy collision as the driver of a car. Your neck pain is constant, severe and radiates down your right arm. On and off you report tingling sensation in the arm.

The candidate will introduce themselves and explain the process of the examination. They will instruct you with actions they wish to perform which may include standing, walking and sitting on the bed. Please follow the candidate's instructions You are allowed to answer their questions before the examination starts.

During the examination you are able to move both arms through a normal range of movement with the exception of restriction of right shoulder movements due to pain. You have good power in the upper limbs and are able to resist the examiner when asked. You have reduced but intact sensation over the outer aspect of the shoulder but otherwise good sensation in the rest of the arms.

2.16 EXAMINATION: Upper Limb Neurology

Task:	Achieved	Not Achieved
Introduces self to the patient and gains consent for examination		
Washes hands or uses alcohol gel		
Explains the examination to the patient and offers a chaperone		
Observes patient from front and behind looking for symmetry of muscle bulk, scars, scoliosis, abnormal hair tufts or evidence spina bifida		
Observes from the side of the patient looking for normal curvature specifically commenting on kyphosis or lordosis		
Ask the patient to sit down and examine tone in both arms		
Tests power in C5 (Shoulder abduction)		
Test power in C6 (Wrist extension)		
Tests power in C7 (Elbow flexion)		
Tests power in C8 (Grip)		
Tests power in T1 Finger abduction)		
Tests reflexes in Elbow flexion, Wrist extension and Hoffman's reflex		
Tests sensation to light touch in C5		
Tests sensation to light touch in C6		
Tests sensation to light touch in C7		
Tests sensation to light touch in C8		
Tests sensation to light touch in T1		
Offers to test pin prick sensation		
Summarises findings and further investigations		
Offers a diagnosis and other differential diagnoses		
Examiner's Global Mark	/5	
Actor's Global Mark	/5	
Total Station Mark	/30	

Learning Points

- General inspection is essential for any physical examination but in particular for the upper limb neurological examination. Check for Scars, Wasting, Involuntary movements, Flickering or Fasciculations and Tremors (SWIFT). This may give you early clues to the overall diagnosis.

- Having a solid core knowledge of the dermatome and myotome map for neurology examination is essential. A good example to follow has been produced by the American Spinal Injury Association

- In the Orthopaedic OSCE stations you are most likely to encounter upper limb pathology with Lower Motor Neuron signs. Ensure you are confident about differentiating between Lower and Upper Motor Neuron signs. Lower Motor Neuron signs are typically reduced tone, weakness and hyporeflexia

2.17 EXAMINATION: Lower Limb Neurology

Candidate's Instructions:

A 60-year-old male patient presents to the emergency department with sudden onset foot drop and foot slapping gait on the right side following a prolonged viral illness.

You are the foundation year doctor in the emergency department and have been asked to perform a neurological examination of his lower limbs then summarize your examination findings back to the examiner.

After 6 minutes the examiner will stop you and ask you to summarise back your findings, suggest your differential diagnoses and your initial management plan.

Examiner's Instructions:

A 60-year-old male patient presents to the emergency department with sudden onset foot drop and foot slapping gait on the right side following a prolonged viral illness.

The candidate is a foundation year doctor in the emergency department and has been asked to perform a neurological examination of his lower limbs.

The station should provide a tendon hammer for reflexes and you are allowed to prompt the candidate to make us of this during the examination.

After 6 minutes stop the candidate whatever stage they are at and ask them to present their findings and suggest relevant investigations and management.

Actor's Instructions:

You are a 60-year-old male patient presenting to the emergency department with sudden onset foot drop and foot slapping gait on the right side following a prolonged viral illness.

The candidate is a foundation year doctor in the emergency department and has been asked to perform a neurological examination of his lower limbs.

During the examination you are able to walk but struggle to control your right foot. When examined on the couch you have weakness in the right foot and ankle and you are unable to lift your foot and ankle to point to your head (dorsiflexion). You have normal sensation.

2.17 EXAMINATION: Lower Limb Neurology

Task:	Achieved	Not Achieved
Introduces self to the patient and gains consent for examination		
Washes hands or uses alcohol gel		
Explains the examination to the patient and offers a chaperone		
Observes patient from front and behind looking for symmetry of muscle bulk, scars, scoliosis, abnormal hair tufts or evidence spina bifida		
Observes from the side of the patient looking for normal curvature specifically commenting on kyphosis or lordosis		
Ask the patient to lie down and examine tone in both legs		
Tests power in L2 (Hip flexion)		
Test power in L3 (Knee extension)		
Tests power in L4 (Ankle dorsiflexion)		
Tests power in L5 (Big toe dorsiflexion/ EHL)		
Tests power in S1 (Ankle plantarflexion)		
Tests reflexes in Knee, Ankle and Babinski response		
Tests sensation to light touch in L2		
Tests sensation to light touch in L3		
Tests sensation to light touch in L4		
Tests sensation to light touch in L5		
Tests sensation to light touch in S1		
Offers to test pin prick sensation		
Summarises findings and further investigations		
Offers a diagnosis and other differential diagnoses		
Examiner's Global Mark	/5	
Actor's Global Mark	/5	
Total Station Mark	/30	

Learning Points

- Having a solid core knowledge of the dermatome and myotome map for neurology examination is essential. A good example to follow has been produced by the American Spinal Injury Association.

- In the Orthopaedic OSCE stations you are most likely to encounter lower limb pathology with Lower Motor Neuron signs. Ensure you are confident about differentiating between Lower and Upper Motor Neuron signs. Lower Motor Neuron signs are typically reduced tone, weakness and hyporeflexia.

- Orthopaedic patients having worn below knee casts for lower limb fractures may cause pressure on the peroneal nerve leading to foot drop.

SKILLS & DATA INTERPRETATION

3.1 SKILLS AND DATA INTERPRETATION: Synovial Fluid Analysis 1

Candidate's Instructions:

A 70-year old male, Mr. John Smith (Hospital No. JS 123456, date of birth 14/04/1946) has been referred by his GP to the Emergency Department with a 3-day history of acute right knee pain and swelling. The patient has tried regular Ibuprofen 200mg TDS with no response and sought medical attention. The knee has been aspirated and the fluid results are available for review.

You are the foundation year doctor and have been asked to review the results and formulate an appropriate management plan. You are provided with adequate information from the patient's pathology reports. Please interpret the results and then summarize your findings to the examiner including further investigations that would aid diagnosis.

You will have 2 minutes to read through the report and then you will be asked a series of questions related to synovial fluid analysis.

Examiner's Instructions:

A 70-year old male, Mr. John Smith (Hospital No. JS 123456, date of birth 14/04/1946) has been referred by his GP to the Emergency Department with a 3-day history of acute right knee pain and swelling. The patient has tried regular Ibuprofen 200mg TDS with no response and sought medical attention. The knee has been aspirated and the fluid results are available for review. He has no past history of joint pain or swelling.

The patient has a significant past medical history of chronic renal impairment, diabetes, hypertension and ischaemic heart disease. His prescription includes amlodipine, ramipril, furosemide, aspirin, simvastatin and metformin. The patient is an ex-smoker and consumes alcohol in excess (over 40 units per week).

The doctor has been asked to interpret the results of the knee synovial fluid aspirate and formulate an appropriate management plan including further investigations that would aid diagnosis.

The candidate will have two minutes to read the information provided on the pathology report. They will be asked to interpret the results and then summarize your findings back to the team. The examiner will ask a series of questions related to synovial fluid analysis.

Questions to ask the candidate:

1. What is the likely cause of Mr. Smith's knee pain?
   Answer – crystal arthritis caused by gout
2. Describe how you would aspirate a knee?
   Answer – the candidate should be able to verbally describe the process of aseptic non-touch technique of knee aspiration
3. What class of drug is allopurinol?
   Answer - Xanthine oxidase inhibitor

4. Assuming this is Mr. Smith's first presentation of gout, when should allopurinol be instituted?

> Answer- After 3 or more attacks of acute gout or if the patient has chronic tophaceous gout. Allopurinol should not be started in the setting of an acute gout flare, but can be continued if a patient was already taking the drug at the time of flare

5. What is the most common bacteriological cause of septic arthritis?

> Answer – Staphylococcus aureus

PATHOLOGY REPORT

Patient Name: John Smith
Patient DOB: 14/04/1946
Patient Age: 70 years
Hospital Number: JS123456

Clinical details: Acute non-traumatic right knee swelling, 3-day history. Unable to weight bear. Difficulty fully flexing or extending knee due to pain. Palpable knee effusion with warmth but no redness. Fluid aspirated. Known renal disease, ischaemic heart disease, hypertension and non-insulin dependent diabetic. Raised CRP 70g/L.

Drug history: amlodipine, ramipril, furosemide, aspirin, simvastatin, metformin

Synovial fluid analysis:

Appearance: Yellow, cloudy fluid.
Cell counts: WCC with neutrophilia
Synovial fluid cytology: Acute inflammatory cells. Multiple needle shaped crystals showing negative birefringence under polarised light microscopy.
Synovial fluid culture: negative gram stain

3.1 SKILLS AND DATA INTERPRETATION: Synovial Fluid Analysis 1

Task:	Achieved	Not Achieved
Confirms patient's name		
Cross references patient's DOB / Hospital number		
States that they would check date of report and check for any addendums and whether report is provisional or final		
Reviews the clinical history and acknowledges the importance of aspiration and synovial fluid analysis		
States clearly to the examiner that there are a number risk factors in Mr Smith's history including; age, alcohol excess, diabetes, diuretic use		
Asks for further investigations including observations and temperature		
States that they would request bloods for WCC, ESR, CRP and plain radiographs of the knee		
Comments on appearance being abnormal and consistent with infection or inflammation		
Comments on white cell count being abnormally high and consistent with infection or inflammation		
Comments on neutrophil count being abnormally high and consistent with infection or inflammation		
Comments on negative microscopy and gram stain suggesting no bacterial infection currently cultured		
Comments on positive crystal microscopy making gout/pseudogout a possible differential		
Comments upon negative bifringence of crystals and therefore gout more likely than pseudogout		
Candidate shows they are aware that septic arthritis and gout/ pseudogout can sometimes co-exist		
Q1. Aware that the likely cause of knee pain is crystal arthritis caused by gout		
Q2. Describes aspiration of the knee using aseptic non-touch technique		

Q3. Knows class of drug of Allopurinol is Xanthine oxidase inhibitor		
Q4. Comments allopurinol should be instituted after 3 or more attacks of acute gout or if the patient has chronic tophaceous gout		
Q5. Aware that most common bacteriological cause of septic arthritis is Staphylococcus aureus		
Summarises findings to examiner		
Answers all questions logically and clearly and presents coherent clinical picture and differential diagnosis	/5	
Examiner's Global Mark	/5	
Total Station Mark	/30	

Learning points:

- Any hot swollen joint must be aspirated if there is any concern about the underlying cause of joint swelling. Fluid should be sent for cytology and microscopy, culture and sensitivity. Knowing characteristic findings of synovial fluid analysis is key.

- Gout is associated with negatively birefringent needle shaped crystals under polarized light microscopy. Pseudogout is related to calcium pyrophosphate crystals which show weak positive birefringence under polarized light microscopy.

- A negative synovial fluid culture does not rule out septic arthritis. If clinical suspicion is in keeping with septic arthritis, the patient should be treated as such. Staphylococcus aureus infection is the most common cause of septic arthritis in adults and children over two.

	Colour	Clarity	Synovial fluid White Cell Count ($x10^6$/L)	Neutrophils (% of total synovial fluid white cell count)	Culture	Crystals	Viscosity
Normal	Clear	Transparent	<200		Negative	None	High
Osteoarthritis	Yellow	Transparent	<2000	<25%	Negative	None	High
Rheumatoid Arthritis	Yellow	Slightly cloudy	>2000	<50%	Negative	None	Low
Gout	Yellow		>2000	<50%	Negative	Urate	Low
Pseudogout	Yellow	Cloudy	>2000	<50%	Negative	Calcium pyrophosphate dihydrate	Low
Septic arthritis	Purulent	Cloudy/Turbid	>50,000	>75%	Often positive	None	Variable

3.2 SKILLS AND DATA INTERPRETATION: Synovial Fluid Analysis 2

Candidate's Instructions:

A 30-year-old man has been admitted with a spontaneous onset painful swollen right knee and a fever. He has no significant post medical history, no trauma to the knee and takes no regular medications. He has had his knee aspirated under aseptic technique.

You are the foundation year doctor and have been asked to review the results and formulate an appropriate management plan. You are provided with adequate information from the patient's pathology reports. Please interpret the results and then summarize your findings to the examiner including further investigations that would aid diagnosis.

You will have 2 minutes to read through the report and then you will be asked a series of questions related to synovial fluid analysis.

Examiner's Instructions:

A 36-year-old man has been admitted with a spontaneous onset painful swollen right knee and a fever. He has no significant post medical history, no trauma to the knee and takes no regular medications. He has had his knee aspirated under aseptic technique.

The results of the analysis are presented below.

The doctor has been asked to interpret the results of the knee synovial fluid aspirate and formulate an appropriate management plan including further investigations that would aid diagnosis.

The candidate will have two minutes to read the information provided on the pathology report. They will be asked to interpret the results and then summarize your findings back to the team. The examiner will ask a series of questions related to synovial fluid analysis.

Questions to ask the candidate:

1.   What is the likely cause of Mr. Whyte's knee pain and what are the general risk factors for this condition?

> Answer – septic arthritis

2.   Describe how you would aspirate a knee?

> Answer – the candidate should be able to verbally describe the process of aseptic non-touch technique of knee aspiration

3.   What would you do next in the context of an acute septic arthritis?

Answer – keep patient nil by mouth for emergency washout in theatre

4.   When should antibiotics be given?

Answer – after a confirmed positive MC&S, ideally from theatre samples unless patient has signs of sepsis or washout delayed

5.   What is the most common bacteriological cause of septic arthritis?

Answer – Staphylococcus aureus

PATHOLOGY REPORT

Patient Name: Barry Whyte
Patient DOB: 16/07/1986
Patient Age: 30 years
Hospital Number: BW456789

Clinical details: Acute non-traumatic right knee swelling. No significant post medical history.

Synovial fluid analysis:

Appearance: Yellow, turbid
Viscosity - High
Cell counts: WCC with neutrophilia
Synovial fluid cytology: Acute inflammatory cells. No crystals
Synovial fluid culture: Gram positive cocci
Glucose level - Low

3.2 SKILLS AND DATA INTERPRETATION: Synovial Fluid Analysis 2

Task:	Achieved	Not Achieved
Confirms patient's name		
Cross references patient's DOB / Hospital number		
States that they would check date of report and check for any addendums and whether report is provisional or final		
Reviews the clinical history and acknowledges the importance of aspiration and synovial fluid analysis		
States clearly to the examiner that the absence of risk factors in a young male trauma or septic arthritis are the likely differentials		
Asks for further investigations including observations and temperature		
States that they would request bloods for WCC, ESR, CRP and plain radiographs of the knee		
Comments on appearance being abnormal and consistent with infection or inflammation		
Comments on white cell count being abnormally high and consistent with infection or inflammation		
Comments on neutrophil count being abnormally high and consistent with infection or inflammation		
Comments on positive microscopy and gram stain suggesting no bacterial infection currently cultured		
Comments on negative crystal microscopy making gout/pseudogout an unlikely differential		
Comments upon low glucose count making bacterial infection possible		
Candidate shows they are aware that septic arthritis and gout/ pseudogout can sometimes co-exist		
Q1. Aware that septic arthritis is the likely diagnosis and gives some risk factors		
Q2. Describes aspiration of the knee using aseptic non-touch technique		
Q3. Describes a further management plan for keeping patient starved ready of washout in theatre		

Q4. Aware that antibiotics should be withheld until MC&S confirmed unless patient has signs of sepsis or washout is delayed		
Q5. Aware that most common bacteriological cause of septic arthritis is staphylococcus aureus		
Summarises findings to examiner		
Answers all questions logically and clearly and presents coherent clinical picture and differential diagnosis	/5	
Examiner's Global Mark	/5	
Total Station Mark	/30	

Learning Points

- Differentiating between infective processes and inflammatory processes on synovial fluid analysis can be challenging. Positive microscopy and Gram stain are highly suggestive of an infective process. Staphylococcus aureus is the most common pathogen in acute bacterial septic arthritis of native joints (i.e. not joint replacements) in adults.

- Septic arthritis is a surgical emergency requiring prompt surgical washout. Without draining the infection cartilage damage is likely to occur within hours causing irreversible joint damage.

- Urate crystals are associated with gout and are needle shaped and demonstrate negative birefringence in polarised light. Calcium pyrophosphate crystals are associated with pseudogout and are rhomboid shaped and demonstrate positive birefringence in polarised light.

	Colour	Clarity	Synovial fluid White Cell Count ($x10^6$/L)	Neutrophils (% of total synovial fluid white cell count)	Culture	Crystals	Viscosity
Normal	Clear	Transparent	<200		Negative	None	High
Osteoarthritis	Yellow	Transparent	<2000	<25%	Negative	None	High
Rheumatoid Arthritis	Yellow	Slightly cloudy	>2000	<50%	Negative	None	Low
Gout	Yellow		>2000	<50%	Negative	Urate	Low
Pseudogout	Yellow	Cloudy	>2000	<50%	Negative	Calcium pyrophosphate dihydrate	Low
Septic arthritis	Purulent	Cloudy /Turbid	>50,000	>75%	Often positive	None	Variable

3.3 SKILLS AND DATA INTERPRETATION: Trauma – Pelvis X-rays

Candidate's Instructions:

An 85-year-old female has been brought into the Emergency Department having been found on the floor by her residential home warden. She has been unable to walk and is complaining of pain in the left hip.

You are the emergency department doctor working in the majors area and have been asked to review the radiographs.

Review the radiographs and present your findings to the examiner along with an appropriate management plan.

There will be questions from the examiner following your presentation.

Examiner's Instructions:

An 85-year-old female has been brought into the ED having been found on the floor by her residential home warden. She has been unable to walk and is complaining of pain in the right hip.

After 6 minutes, please stop the candidate and ask: "Please summarise your findings and discuss how you would like to investigate and manage this patient."

X Ray Review:

Assume the radiographs have the complete patient identifiers and date they were taken.

They are technically adequate with an AP projection of both hips including the proximal femurs and both iliac crests and a lateral projection of the left hip. There is no excessive rotation and the penetration is acceptable.

The most obvious abnormality is a left displaced intracapsular neck of femur fracture. Joint space is maintained, and all other joints are appropriately aligned. There are no soft tissue abnormalities and no other fractures identified on reviewing the cortical outline of all the bones.

Questions;

1. What is the most common cause of fragility fractures?
Osteoporosis

2. Which arteries contribute blood supply to the femoral head?
a.   Medial circumflex femoral artery (main contributor)
b.   Lateral circumflex femoral artery
c.   Inferior Gluteal artery
d.   Superior gluteal artery

e. Artery of Ligamentum Teres (patent in children, minimal supply in adults)

3. What is the main concern with intracapsular fractures?

Loss of blood supply to the femoral head

4. How should intracapsular fractures be treated in the older population?

Arthroplasty (hemiarthroplasty or total hip replacement)

5. How should extracapsular fractures be treated?

Fixation with dynamic hip screw or intramedullary nailing

Image for interpretation

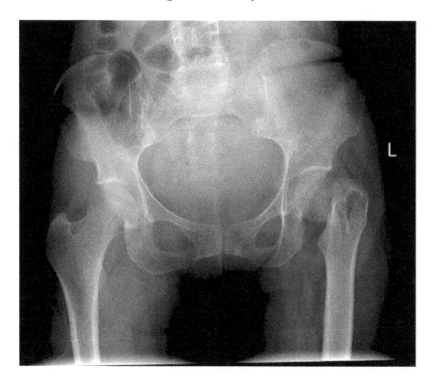

3.3 SKILLS AND DATA INTERPRETATION: Trauma – Pelvis X-rays

Task:	Achieved	Not Achieved
States that they would confirm patient's name		
States that they would confirm patient's DOB/ hospital number		
States that they would confirm date of the radiograph		
Identifies AP of pelvis		
Identifies lateral of left hip		
Comments on rotation		
Comments on adequacy		
Comments on penetration		
Identifies fracture of left neck of femur		
Identifies that this is a displaced fracture		
Identifies that this is an intracapsular fracture		
Comments on bone and joint alignment		
Comments on joint space of the hip		
Comments on cortical outline of all bones to exclude other injury		
Comments on soft tissues		
Demonstrates understanding of need for urgent orthopaedic referral		
Suggests examination of joints above and below		
Suggests need for medical clearance for underlying cause of fall		
Demonstrates understanding of need for surgery		
Summarises findings to examiner		
Answers all questions logically and clearly	/5	
Examiner's Global Mark	/5	
Total Station Mark	/30	

Learning Points

- Reviewing two different views of any injury is essential – subtle fractures may only be easily identified on one of the views.

- Even if there is an obvious fracture or abnormality, ensure you systematically assess the rest of the radiograph to avoid missing other abnormalities.

- Displaced intracapsular neck of femur fractures in the elderly are serious injuries with a high risk of non-union and avascular necrosis – they are usually managed with urgent surgery in the form of a hemiarthroplasty or a total hip replacement.

3.4 SKILLS AND DATA INTERPRETATION: Metabolic bone profile

Candidate's Instructions:

You are a foundation year doctor currently working in rheumatology and help with the weekly metabolic bone clinic. A new clinical nurse specialist has just started working with the team. She has seen a complicated patient in clinic and would like to discuss the blood results. The consultant is not around and she has asked for your advice. Please discuss the results with her and help come up with an appropriate management plan.

Mr David West
DW987654
DOB; 17/7/40

The results are below with reference ranges in brackets:

Sodium (Na+)	136mmol/L (135-145mmol/L)
Potassium (K+)	4.6mmol/L (3.5-5.0mmol/L)
Creatinine(Creat)	670µmol/L (71-115 µmol/L)
Calcium (Ca++)	2.21mmol/L (2.15-2.6mmol/L)
Albumin	40g/L (35-50g/L)
Alkaline phosphatase (ALP)	293 IU/L (30-130 IU/L)
Phosphate	2.06mmol/L (0.8-1.4mmol/L)
PTH	1050 ng/L (10-70ng/L)

Examiner's Instructions:

A patient with known kidney disease and non-specific joint pains has been referred to the metabolic bone clinic. They were seen in the clinic yesterday by the new clinical nurse specialist along with the consultant. Several investigations were requested and the results are now available. The consultant is not around and the nurse specialist would like to discuss the results with another member of the team.

The results show secondary hyperparathyroidism in a patient with known end stage renal failure. It is not primary or tertiary hyperparathyroidism because the calcium level is low.

Actor's Instructions:

You are a new CNS working with the metabolic bone team. You saw a complex patient yesterday in clinic and discussed him with the consultant at the time. The consultant suggested that send off a few investigations. You now have the results but are not entirely sure how best to interpret them. The consultant is on leave but another member of the medical team is around to provide advice.

The patient has known end stage renal failure and is on peritoneal dialysis. They have had some mild non-specific generalised aches and pains recently but no evidence of arthritis.

You have several questions for the doctor

1. What is the likely diagnosis?
2. Would calcium supplements be helpful
3. Should you give them vitamin D supplements and if so which kind
4. Are there any other types of drugs that could be helpful?
5. If drugs don't work what would be the next step

The appropriate answers should be:

1. Secondary hyperparathyroidism in a patient with known end stage renal failure
2. Start a phosphate binder – usually calcium supplements such as calcichew
3. Treat with a vitamin D analogue (alfacalcidol or calcitriol) – the candidate must ensure that they specify the right kind of vitamin D preparation
4. Consider a calcimimetic drug (cinacalcet)
5. If the above isn't working, consider referral to endocrine surgeon for parathyroidectomy

3.4 SKILLS AND DATA INTERPRETATION: Metabolic bone profile

Task:	Achieved	Not Achieved
Introduces him/herself to the CNS		
Elicits the current situation		
Elicits the concerns of the CNS		
States that they would confirm patient's name		
States that they would confirm patient's DOB/ hospital number		
States that they would confirm date of the blood test results		
Identifies raised creatinine consistent with renal failure		
Checks and confirms normal Na+ and K+		
Identifies abnormally high PTH level		
Identifies high ALP		
Identifies high phosphate and normal Ca++ levels		
Gives the correct diagnosis – secondary hyperparathyroidism		
Identifies that this is due to the underlying renal failure		
Correctly identifies that calcium supplements would be useful		
Agrees that vitamin D supplementation should be given		
Identifies the correct form of vitamin D replacement – alfacalcidol		
Suggests the use of cinacalcet		
Advises that parathyroid surgery may be required if the patient fails to respond to the above measures		
Agrees a plan of action with the nurse specialist		
Summarises appropriately		
Examiner's Global Mark	/5	
Actor's Global Mark	/5	
Total Station Mark	/30	

Learning Points

- In end stage renal failure replacement of correction of vitamin D with conventional preparations of cholecalciferol or ergocalciferol will not work as these preparations require hydroxylation in the kidney to become active. Alfacalcidol or calcitriol should be used instead.

- If untreated patients can develop tertiary hyperparathyroidism in end stage renal failure and hypercalcaemia will develop.

- Cinacalcet can lead to hypocalcaemia it is important to repeat the bone biochemistry readings after starting it and adjust the dose accordingly.

3.5 SKILLS AND DATA INTERPRETATION:
Scrubbing and gowning

Candidate's Instructions:

You are the foundation year doctor on the orthopaedic team. You have been called to theatre to assist in a total hip replacement surgery.

Scrub up and put on a gown and surgical gloves.

Following this there will be some questions from the examiner.

Examiner's Instructions:

The candidate is required to demonstrate scrubbing up technique and appropriate donning of a gown and gloves.

A sink with appropriate taps, surgical brush and surgical scrub are provided. A packed surgical gown and towels are provided as are appropriately sized packed sterile gloves.

You will finish by asking the candidate the following questions:

1. Which patient allergy group should be identified and acted upon before theatre management?
a.   Latex allergy, some hospitals still use latex containing surgical gloves

2. Once scrubbed up – which parts of your gown and gloves can be considered sterile?
a. Hand to elbow and nipple to mid-waist only

3. What is sterilisation?
a. A process of removal or deactivation of micro-organisms from a surface including bacteria, fungi and viruses

4. What types of sterilisation do you know?
a. Heat sterilisation, Chemical sterilisation, Radiation sterilization

5. What steps would you take in you sustained a needlestick injury?
a. Expose the wound and thoroughly irrigate encouraging bleeding. Document injury and inform line manager/ theatre manager. Attend Occupational Health or ED for further management according to local Trust policies.

Actor's Instructions:

No actor is required for this station

3.5 SKILLS AND DATA INTERPRETATION: Scrubbing and gowning

Task:	Achieved	Not Achieved
Opens gown pack using appropriate technique		
Opens gloves onto sterile field using appropriate technique		
Puts on surgical mask		
Turns on taps and checks flow and temperature		
Uses scrubbing brush to clean under nails		
Applies appropriate volume of scrub solution		
Scrubs palm to palm		
Scrubs palm to dorsum each side		
Scrubs backs of fingers to palms with interlocked fingers		
Scrubs bases of thumbs		
Scrubs fingertips to palms		
Scrubs both wrists		
Scrubs both forearms		
Turns off taps using elbows		
Appropriate drying technique		
Picks up gown appropriately and puts arms into sleeves without revealing hands		
Dons gloves using closed or open technique		
Scrubs for appropriate time		
Keeps fingers above elbows at all points		
Avoids touching anything non-sterile throughout		
Answers all questions logically and clearly	/5	
Examiner's Global Mark	/5	
Total Station Mark	/30	

Learning Points

- The first scrub of an operating list should be at least five minutes long. Further scrubs between cases can be shorter – around three minutes.

- If at any point during the scrubbing process the hands or forearms come into contact with anything non-sterile then the entire process must be restarted from the beginning

- Double gloving is commonplace in orthopaedic operating theatres – the risk of a glove perforation is high and two layers reduces the risks of contamination to both patient and surgeon.

3.6 SKILLS AND DATA INTERPRETATION: Cervical spine immobilisation

Candidate's Instructions:

A 25-year-old walks into the Emergency Department shortly after being involved in a road traffic accident resulting in him being thrown from his motorcycle. He is complaining of neck pain.

The patient has been taken to the resuscitation area of the ED and a trauma call declared. You are the orthopaedic foundation year doctor and have been asked to immobilise the patient's cervical spine.

Another member of the trauma team is available to assist you if required.

Examiner's Instructions:

A 25-year-old motorcyclist has attended the ED shortly after being involved in a road traffic accident resulting in him coming off his motorcycle. He has removed his own helmet and walked at the scene. He has self-presented to the ED complaining of neck pain. He has been transferred to the resuscitation area and is standing up next to the bed.

The orthopaedic foundation year doctor on call has been asked to immobilise the patient's cervical spine.

A stiff cervical spine collar, blocks and a Velcro strap/tape is provided. A third person is available to assist in providing in line immobilisation if requested by the candidate.

Actor's Instructions:

You are a 25-year-old fit and well man involved in a road traffic accident whilst riding your motorcycle. You were thrown from the bike and managed to get up yourself at the scene. You have walked since the accident and have taken off your own helmet. You have walked into the Emergency Department as you have a painful neck. You do not have any symptoms of numbness or weakness in any of your limbs and no other parts of your body are painful. You have been brought through to the resuscitation area of the ED and are standing next to the bed holding your neck.

You know where you are, the time and are not confused. You recall all the events surrounding the accident. You are not combative and comply with the candidate's instructions.

Assistant's Instructions:

You are not to provide any advice to the candidate. If the candidate requests that you manually immobilise the patient's neck then you are to place one hand on either side of the patient's head with your fingers touching the shoulders holding the head in a stable position. You are to maintain this position until asked to stop by the candidate.

3.6 SKILLS AND DATA INTERPRETATION: Cervical spine immobilisation

Task:	Achieved	Not Achieved
Introduces self		
Clarifies patient's name		
Checks name and expertise of assistance		
Puts of gloves/apron		
Asks patient to lie on bed		
Holds patient's head in neutral position		
Requests assistance from assistant to hold head		
Measures size of collar using fingers from lower chin to trapezius		
Adjusts cervical collar to appropriate size		
Slides collar under neck		
Closes collar applying appropriate tension		
Asks if patient is comfortable		
Applies blocks to sides of patient's head		
Applies tape/Velcro strap to immobilise head with blocks		
Ensures assistant applying in line immobilisation until blocks and tape applied		
Advises patient that collar will need to remain until injury has been excluded		
Organises Xray in timely manner to minimise time in collar		
Confident manner with patient		
Remains calm		
Appropriate communication with assistant		
Examiner's Global Mark	/5	
Actor's Global Mark	/5	
Total Station Mark	/30	

Learning Points

- Even if a patient has walked away from an accident they could still have significant neck injuries and require cervical spine immobilisation until an injury can be excluded. The NICE guidelines can guide on which patients require plain film imaging and immobilisation.

- Safe application of a cervical spine immobilisation collar requires teamwork with one team member applying manual in line immobilisation whilst another sizes and applies the collar.

- The first line investigation of a patient with a painful neck following significant trauma would be a CT scan as this is less likely to miss subtle injuries and is readily available in most hospitals now. The NICE Head and neck injury guidelines exist to advise clinicians on the criteria for higher imaging.

3.7 SKILLS AND DATA INTERPRETATION: ATLS
Primary survey and skills

Candidate's Instructions:

A 56-year-old man has been brought by ambulance to the Emergency Department following falling from a ladder at a height of 3m.

You are the orthopaedic foundation year doctor in the trauma team and a primary survey has been completed. Please describe and demonstrate on a model the methods airway maintenance in trauma, describe emergency airway techniques and demonstrate decompression of a tension pneumothorax.

Examiner's Instructions:

A 56-year-old man has been brought by ambulance to the Emergency Department following falling from a ladder at a height of 3m. A primary survey is in progress and the candidate has been asked to describe airway maintenance including emergency airway options and decompression of a tension pneumothorax.

During this station there will be no actor, the candidate will use a model to demonstrate their skills and follow this up with discussion point with you as the examiner.

Actor's Instructions:

Model used for demonstration purposes in this station which facilitates further discussion between candidate and examiner

3.7 SKILLS AND DATA INTERPRETATION: ATLS Primary survey and skills

Task:	Achieved	Not Achieved
Introduces self to team and patient		
Washes hands/uses alcohol gel		
Puts on gown and gloves		
Ensures C spine is controlled with in line immobilisation or collar and blocks		
Assesses airway - look listens and feels		
Airway manoeuvres - jaw thrust if c spine concern		
Describes signs of impending airway problems		
Safely delivers oxygen and high flow		
Able to insert airway adjuncts if needed		
Aware that NPA not suitable if potential for base of skull fracture		
Demonstrates examination of the trachea and chest with baseline obs		
Describes signs of tension pneumothorax - reduced air entry, reduced chest expansion, hyper resonant percussion note		
Aware that tracheal deviation is a late sign		
Thoracocentesis - Inserts large bore cannula 2nd ICS MCL		
Reassess chest for improvement after intervention		
Monitors cannula to ensure it doesn't occlude and cause reaccumulation of tension PTX		
States would fully reassess the patient at this point - Rpt ABC and		
Aware for need of a definitive chest drain		
Describes need for CXR as part of primary survey		
Avoids focusing on distracting injury of painful feet		
Remains confident and calm		
Examiner's Global Mark	/5	
Total Station Mark	/30	

Learning Points

- This station is about being safe and sticking to the principles of ABC. This stepwise approach ensures that you can diagnose and treat immediately life-threatening conditions in the most urgent order. Don't remain focused on airway management if you are unable to maintain it and always state that you would request anaesthetic assistance

- Once you have delivered a treatment eg; decompressed a tension pneumothorax it is good practice to re-start your assessment from A – Airway again and assess for change in the patient's state

- You may have a helper on this station with you, prepare in advance a series of requests that you might have at each checkpoint eg; high flow oxygen at A, sats probe at B and a cannula and blood tests at C.

3.8 SKILLS AND DATA INTERPRETATION: VTE Risk assessment

Candidate's Instructions:

A 74-year-old female patient is being admitted for a planned total hip replacement operation which is due to start at 0900.

You are the orthopaedic foundation year doctor and have been asked to assess the patient's risk of thromboembolism and prescribe appropriate prophylaxis. You are not required to examine the patient.

You have 6 minutes to consider the risk factors and prescribe on the drug chart. Following this the examiner will ask some questions.

Examiner's Instructions:

A 74-year-old female patient is being admitted for a planned total hip replacement operation.

The candidate is required to assess the patient's risk of thromboembolism and prescribe appropriate prophylaxis.

If asked appropriate questions the actor will provide all the required information to allow a complete assessment.

A blank drug chart is provided.

After 6 minutes the candidate should be directed to complete the drug chart if not yet started. Ask the candidate for how long they would continue the patient's pharmacological thromboprophylaxis on discharge.

Actor's Instructions:

You are a 74-year-old with a 3-year history of worsening left hip pain and have attended the hospital to be admitted for a planned left total hip replacement.

You weigh 59kg. You have had a right total knee replacement 4 years ago without any perioperative issues. You have no known drug allergies. You take Ramipril 2.5mg OD and simvastatin 20mg OD and have done for 7 years. Your blood pressure is well controlled. Other than your high blood pressure you do not have any other medical problems or symptoms. You have never had any problems with your kidneys and you were told at your preoperative assessment that your kidney blood tests were normal (as were all your other blood tests).

You have never had a deep vein thrombosis. Your brother had a deep vein thrombosis following his hip replacement 4 years ago. He needed to have blood thinning medication for six months and has had no issues since.

You smoked 10 cigarettes a day from age 40 to 55, and have not smoked since age 55.

You have not had any recent falls and no issues with excessive bleeding. You have never had varicose veins nor any problems with the blood supply to your legs and feet.

3.8 SKILLS AND DATA INTERPRETATION: VTE Risk assessment

Task:	Achieved	Not Achieved
Introduces self		
Checks patient's name and DOB		
Explains to patient reason for interaction		
Confirms procedure patient is undergoing		
Asks about drug allergies		
Asks about current medications		
Asks patient's weight		
Asks about past medical history including renal problems		
Asks about previous personal history of thromboembolic disease		
Asks about previous family history of thromboembolic disease		
Asks smoking history		
Asks about bleeding risks – e.g. falls		
Asks about contraindications to anti-embolic stockings (AES) – e.g. problems with vascular supply to legs		
Documents patient's allergy status		
Documents patient's weight		
Prescribes appropriate low molecular weight heparin or Factor Xa inhibitor		
Prescribes first dose on evening of surgery		
Prescribes bilateral anti-embolic stockings (AES)		
Aware of guideline for pharmacological thromboprophylaxis for 28 days post operation.		
Summaries appropriately and answers questions		
Examiner's Global Mark	/5	
Actor's Global Mark	/5	
Total Station Mark	/30	

Learning Points

- Total hip replacement surgery is associated with a high risk of venous thromboembolism. All patients undergoing THR should receive extended chemoprophylaxis and TEDS unless contraindicated

- Though not a drug, anti-embolic stockings must be prescribed on the patient's drug chart

- Factor Xa inhibitors (eg Rivaroxaban) are increasing in popularity for postoperative thromboprophylaxis. They can be taken orally as opposed to low molecular weight heparin which is given as a subcutaneous injection. Uncontrolled bleeding can be a problem with factor Xa inhibitors as no reliable method of reversal is currently available.

EMERGENCY CASES

4.1 EMERGENCY CASES: Ward – Compartment Syndrome

Candidate's instructions

You are the SHO on call overnight in a busy DGH. You are called to see a young male patient who has undergone tibial nailing today for a closed NV intact tibial shaft fracture. The nurses are concerned that they can't keep him comfortable and have asked you for more analgesia.

Your brief assessment can include a short focused history, examinations for key signs and will include radiograph interpretation.

There will be some questions from the examiner following this.

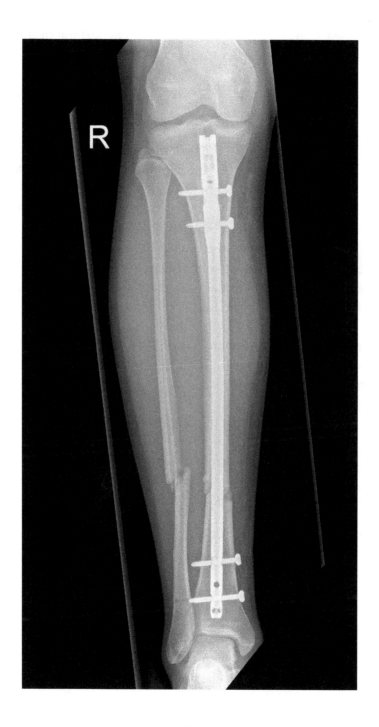

Examiner's instructions

This is a case of postoperative compartment syndrome of the leg following tibial nailing earlier today.

Ask the candidate to assess the patient including brief history, examination and management.

Once the assessment shows that the patient has had high levels of opioid analgesia without relief the candidate should state that they are considering compartment syndrome. Candidate should recognise the need for urgent surgical decompression. During the assessment the candidate will examine the limb and when performing appropriate tests you will offer the positive findings of tense compartments, severe tenderness and worsening pain on passive stretch. The limb remain perfused with a palpable pulse but reduced sensation in the foot.

You should allow the candidate 6 minute for assessment and then a further 2 minutes to present their findings and management plan and answer your questions.

You should ask the following questions;

1. What is the definition of compartment syndrome?
2. What are the signs of a compartment syndrome?
3. Describe the underlying pathology of compartment syndrome?
4. Outline the main management points in the BOAST guideline for compartment syndrome?

Actor's instructions

You are in extreme pain following an operation on your tibial fracture earlier today. The pain is the worst you've ever felt and you are getting pins and needles in the leg. You have had lots of extra morphine pain relief without success.

The candidate will ask some basic questions then proceed to examine your leg. Due to the nature of the condition the examiners will feedback the positive findings to the candidate.

4.1 EMERGENCY CASES: Ward – Compartment Syndrome

Task:	Achieved	Not Achieved
Describes ABC approach to patient assessment		
Establishes the background of tibial nailing for a closed fracture earlier today		
Elicits the chronicity and progression of pain		
Elicits the severity of pain		
Assesses the previous use of analgesia and recognises high levels of opioid have failed to control pain		
Asks about neurovascular symptoms including tingling, pins and needles or numbness		
Recognises the potential for compartment syndrome and states the terminology		
States an initial plan of high elevation, release of plaster cast and analgesia		
States signs to observe on examination eg; patient in extremis, severe swelling of the limb, pale limb in advanced compartment syndrome		
Offers examination of the affected limb including neurovascular examination		
Demonstrates palpation of the limb to elicit tense compartments (cues given by the examiner)		
Demonstrates assessment of pain on passive stretch of the anterior compartment of the leg		
Demonstrates assessment of pain on passive stretch of the deep and superficial posterior compartment of the leg		
Demonstrates assessment of neurovascular status of the limb		
Recognises need for urgent surgical decompression recommends patient kept nil by mouth		
States would contact senior team, anaesthetist and book patient onto emergency theatre list		
Candidate defines compartment syndrome when asked		
Candidate states the signs of compartment syndrome as tense compartment with pain, exacerbation on passive stretch, paraesthesia, pallor, pulselessness, paralysis		

Able to state the underlying problem in compartment syndrome		
Able to outline the BOAST protocol for management of compartment syndrome		
Examiner's Global Mark	/5	
Actor's Global Mark	/5	
Total Station Mark	/30	

Learning Points

• The British Orthopaedic Association have produced guidelines for diagnosis and management of compartment syndrome under their BOAST series. The following are selected key guidelines that are important to consider in the OSCE scenario and clinical practice;

• Assessment for compartment syndrome should be routine after significant injury or surgery to a limb.

• Key clinical findings are pain out of proportion to the injury and pain on pain passive movement of the muscles within the affected compartment.

• Compartment syndrome is an emergency and operation should be performed within 1 hour of the decision to operate.

Further information can be found at:
https://www.boa.ac.uk/wp-content/uploads/2014/12/BOAST-10.pdf

4.2 EMERGENCY CASES: ED – Open Fracture Management

Candidate's instructions

You are on the trauma team at the major trauma centre for the area. A young adult male, not yet identified, has been brought in by HEMS following RTA. He has multiple injuries including a tibial shaft fracture with a large contaminated open wound. There is considerable skin loss and fat, muscle and bone is visible.

Your brief assessment can include a short focused history, examinations for key signs and will include radiograph interpretation.

There will be some questions from the examiner following this.

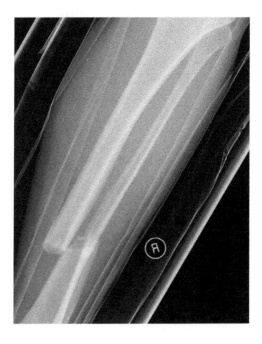

Examiner's instructions

The candidate is on the trauma team at the major trauma centre for the area. A young adult male, not yet identified, has been brought in by HEMS following RTA. He has multiple injuries including a tibial shaft fracture with a large contaminated open wound. There is considerable skin loss and fat, muscle and bone is visible.

Ask the candidate to describe their initial management approach to this scenario which should be guided by ATLS protocol.

Following a satisfactory answer please ask the candidate to now focus on the open fracture management. Candidate should recognise the need for antibiotics, tetanus and urgent surgical debridement.

You should allow the candidate 6 minute for assessment and then a further 2 minutes to present their findings and management plan and answer your questions.

1. Describe a classification system for open fractures?
2. Describe the key points of the BOAST guidelines for management of open fractures?

What is the indication for immediate out of hours debridement?

Actor's instructions

You have been involved in an RTA. The candidate will describe to the examiner with demonstration steps to assess your injuries. You do not need to do anything to assist this scenario.

The candidate will ask some basic questions then proceed to examine your leg. Due to the nature of the condition the examiners will feedback the positive findings to the candidate.

Mark scheme– Open Fracture Management

Task:	Achieved	Not Achieved
Introduces self to the patient and gains consent for examination		
Washes hands or uses alcohol gel		
Recognises the mechanism of injury warrants major trauma centre management		
Describes ATLS approach to primary survey		
States that airway should be assessed and inline c-spine immobilisation maintained		
States that thoracic trauma should assessed		
States that circulation including major source of bleeding should be assess eg, abdomen, pelvis and long bones		
Describes safe resuscitation of the patient including oxygen, analgesia, fluids +/- transfusion		
States that bloods including group and save and cross match should be taken along with radiographs of the chest and pelvis		
Able to describe the radiograph of a tibial fracture		
Able to describe appearance of an open wound		
Describes appropriate examination of the affected limb for neurovascular status		
Correctly identifies this as an open tibial fracture and recognises the importance in management of these injuries		
Describes the need of temporary wound coverage with saline and gauze followed by splinting		
Recognises need for administration of antibiotics and tetanus		
Recognises need for urgent surgical debridement		
Summarises situation to the examiner		
Candidate is able to describe the Gustilo Anderson Classification for open fractures		
Able to outline the BOAST protocol for management of open fractures		
States the indications for immediate out of hours surgery as neurovascular injury or gross contamination eg; farm waste		
Actor's Global Mark	/5	
Examiner's Global Mark	/5	
Total Station Mark	/30	

Learning Points

The British Orthopaedic Association have produced guidelines for diagnosis and management of open fractures under their BOAST series. The following are selected key guidelines that are important to consider in the OSCE scenario and clinical practice;

- Administration of antibiotics

- Any vascular impairment should be treated within 3-4 hours

- Definitive management should be performed in a trauma centre with the input of multiple disciplines including plastic surgery

Gustilo Grade	Definition
I	Open fracture, clean wound, wound <1 cm in length
II	Open fracture, wound > 1 cm but < 10 cm in length without extensive soft-tissue damage, flaps, avulsions
III	Open fracture with extensive soft-tissue laceration, damage, or loss or an open segmental fracture. Any open fractures caused by farm injuries are Type II
IIIA	Type III fracture with adequate periosteal coverage of the fracture bone despite the extensive soft-tissue laceration or damage
IIIB	Type III fracture with extensive soft-tissue loss and periosteal stripping and bone damage
IIIC	Type III fracture associated with an arterial injury requiring repair

Further information can be found at:
http://www.boa.ac.uk/publications/boast-4-the-management-of-sever-open-lower-limb-fractures/

4.3 EMERGENCY CASES: ED – Neurovascular Injury

Candidate's instructions

A 19-year-old man is brought into the emergency department by the police. You have been informed he has been stabbed in his arm approximately 2 hours ago. He is complaining his hand feels cold and numb.

You are the foundation year 2 doctor in accident and emergency who has been asked to assess him and report your findings and management plan to your consultant. Your brief assessment can include a short focused history, examinations for key signs.

Once you approach the patient you see that he has sustained a deep laceration to the antecubital fossa.

There will be some questions from the examiner following this.

Examiner's instructions

A 19-year-old man is brought into the emergency department by the police. You have been informed he has been stabbed in his arm approximately 2 hours ago. He is complaining his hand feels cold and numb.

The candidate is a foundation year 2 doctor in ED who has been asked to assess him and report their findings and management plan to their consultant. When they go to see the patient, you are presented with a deep laceration to the antecubital fossa.

The patient has no median nerve function, no radial pulse and a cold hand.

You should allow the candidate 6 minute for assessment and then a further 2 minutes to present their findings and management plan and answer your questions.

1. What are the signs of a vascular injury?
2. What are the signs of a radial nerve injury?
3. What are the signs of a median nerve injury?
4. What are the signs of an ulnar nerve injury?
5. When should a neurovascular injury be treated?

Actor's instructions

You are a 19 year old man who has been stabbed in the arm 2 hours ago. You can report to the candidate that you have felt that the affected hand is cold and numb to the touch.

The candidate will ask some basic questions then proceed to examine your leg. Due to the nature of the condition the examiners will feedback the positive findings to the candidate.

4.3 EMERGENCY CASES: ED – Neurovascular Injury

Task:	Achieved	Not Achieved
Describes ABC approach to patient assessment		
Establishes the background injury		
Elicits the timing of injury		
Elicits the severity of pain		
Asks about neurovascular symptoms including tingling, pins and needles, numbness, weakness		
Recognises the potential for neurovascular injury		
States signs to observe on examination eg; position of wound, pallor of limb, lack of movement		
Offers examination of the affected limb including neurovascular examination		
Demonstrates palpation of the limb to elicit temperature difference or tense compartments		
Demonstrates assessment distal pulses eg; radial and ulnar artery		
Demonstrates assessment of capillary refill time		
Demonstrates assessment of neurological function		
Recognises need for urgent surgical intervention		
States would contact senior team, anaesthetist and book patient onto emergency theatre list		
Candidate states the signs vascular injury when asked		
Able to describe signs of radial nerve injury		
Able to describe signs of median nerve injury		
Able to describe signs of ulnar nerve injury		
Describes 'ischaemia' time and urgency of repair within 4 hours		
Summarises the situation to the examiner		
Examiner's Global Mark	/5	
Actor's Global Mark	/5	
Total Station Mark	/30	

Learning Points

- Anatomical knowledge of the area of injury can guide examination and management. Gauging the direction of injury and the weapon can also help.

- Detailed neurovascular examination with clear documentation is important and referral onto specialty services will require this.

- Ischaemia time of four hours is the approximate cut off where tissue begins to become non-viable. Thus, it is important to know the time of injury as it may guide surgical intervention.

4.4 EMERGENCY CASES: ED – Shoulder Dislocation

Candidate's instructions

A 25-year old man attends the emergency department following a fall. He is complaining about excruciating pain and that his shoulder now looks 'odd'.

You are the foundation year doctor working in ED who has been asked to assess him. Your brief assessment can include a short focused history, examinations for key signs and will include radiograph interpretation.

There will be some questions from the examiner following this.

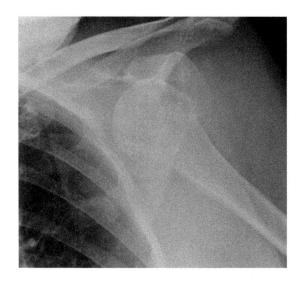

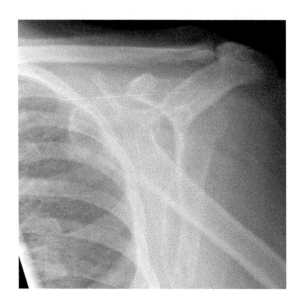

Examiner's instructions

A 25-year old man attends the emergency department following a fall. He is complaining about excruciating pain and that his shoulder now looks 'odd'.

The foundation year doctor working in the emergency department has been asked to assess him. They have taken a history and examination and reviewed the plain radiographs which show an anterior shoulder dislocation.

You should allow the candidate 6 minute for assessment and then a further 2 minutes to present their findings and management plan and answer your questions.

1. What is the difference in presentation and radiographic findings between anterior and posterior dislocation of the shoulder?
2. Which nerve is particularly at risk during anterior shoulder dislocation?
3. Describe the innervation of the axillary nerve?
4. Describe two lesions which may occur during repeat dislocations?
5. Name the nerve root contributing to the brachial plexus and which cord gives rise to the axillary nerve?

Actor's instructions

You are a 25 year old man who has has attended the emergency department after a fall. Your shoulder is painful and you have notices that it appears 'odd'.

The candidate will ask some basic questions then proceed to examine your leg. Due to the nature of the condition the examiners will feedback the positive findings to the candidate.

4.4 EMERGENCY CASES: ED – Shoulder Dislocation

Task:	Achieved	Not Achieved
Describes ABC approach to patient assessment		
Establishes the background injury and whether there were any previous episodes		
Elicits the timing of injury		
Elicits the severity of pain		
Asks about neurovascular symptoms including tingling, pins and needles, numbness, weakness		
Offers examination of the affected limb including neurovascular examination		
States signs to observe on examination eg; sulcus sign, flat deltoid		
Demonstrates testing sensation over regimental badge distribution		
Demonstrates assessment distal pulses eg; radial and ulnar artery		
Demonstrates assessment of capillary refill time		
Demonstrates assessment of neurological function		
When shown the radiograph establishes the diagnosis of anterior shoulder dislocation		
Recognises need for analgesia and urgent reduction		
States would attempt reduction under sedation or contact anaesthetist and book patient onto emergency theatre list		
Able to describe the difference between anterior and posterior dislocation of the shoulder		
Able to describe the axillary nerve is at risk during dislocation		
Able to describe that the axillary nerve innervates deltoid and teres minor and the regimental badge distribution of sensation		
Able to describe a Hill Sachs lesion or Bankart lesion		
Able name the nerve roots forming the brachial plexus and the axillary nerve arises from the posterior cord		
Summarises the situation to the examiner		
Examiner's Global Mark	/5	
Actor's Global Mark	/5	
Total Station Mark	/30	

Learning Points

- Deciphering between anterior and posterior dislocations is key in good quality management as different reduction techniques will be appropriate for one type rather than the other. Examination and good plain radiograph interpretation are key to this. Posterior dislocation of the shoulder is rare and can be associated with abnormal mechanisms of injury such as electric shock or seizures. The classic description of the posterior dislocation of the humeral head is the 'light bulb' appearance.

- Neurological examination is important, axillary nerve is at risk and knowing the motor and sensory innervation of this nerve is important. Use this scenario to read up and learn the brachial plexus which is a common exam question

- Management strategies are either closed reduction in the emergency department or theatre and it would be useful to familiarise yourself with some methods such as Kocher's or Stimpson's. Very rarely open reduction in theatre will be necessary.

4.5 EMERGENCY CASES: Ward - Hip Dislocation

Candidate's instructions

A 70-year old woman has fallen on the ward and is now complaining about pain in her hip. The day foundation year doctor had organised an X-ray of the hip but not managed to review the patient. She has recently undergone a total hip replacement and is now three days post-op.

You are the foundation year doctor working on the wards overnight who has been asked to assess her. Your brief assessment can include a short focused history, examinations for key signs and will include radiograph interpretation.

There will be some questions from the examiner following this.

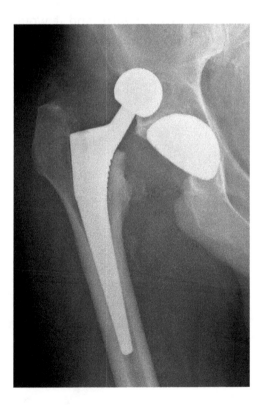

Examiner's instructions

A 70-year old woman has fallen on the ward and is now complaining about pain in her hip. The day foundation year doctor had organised an X-ray of the hip but not managed to review the patient. She has recently undergone a total hip replacement and is now three days post-op.

The candidate is a foundation year doctor working on the wards overnight who has been asked to assess her. They have taken a history and examination and the plain radiographs show a dislocated total hip replacement.

Ask the candidate to describe the x-ray. Ask the candidate how they would assess the patient. There should be a systematic approach to the history and examination. An ABC approach to rule out any immediate problems. These are all within normal parameters. They should offer information about ruling out a head injury and looking at the observations. None of these are out of range.

You should allow the candidate 6 minute for assessment and then a further 2 minutes to present their findings and management plan and answer your questions.

You should ask the following questions;

1. What is the difference in presentation and radiographic findings between anterior and posterior dislocation of the hip?
2. Which nerve is particularly at risk during posterior hip dislocation?
3. Describe a motor and a sensory sign you might see with sciatic nerve injury?
4. Describe two main branches of the sciatic nerve?
5. What further intervention may be needed in a patient with recurrent dislocations of a total hip replacement

Actor's instructions

You are a 70 year old lady who is recovering following a total hip replacement operation 3 days ago. You have fallen on the ward and have a painful hip and you are unable to walk.

The candidate will ask some basic questions then proceed to examine your leg. Due to the nature of the condition the examiners will feedback the positive findings to the candidate.

4.5 EMERGENCY CASES: Ward - Hip Dislocation

Task:	Achieved	Not Achieved
Describes ABC approach to patient assessment		
Establishes the background operation and whether there were any previous episodes		
Elicits the timing of injury		
Elicits the severity of pain		
Asks about neurovascular symptoms including tingling, pins and needles, numbness, weakness		
Offers examination of the affected limb including neurovascular examination		
States signs to observe on examination eg; shortened, internally rotation leg		
Demonstrates assessing gross sensory function		
Demonstrates assessing gross motor function		
Demonstrates assessment of capillary refill time		
Demonstrates assessment of distal pulses at posterior tibial and dorsalis pedis artery		
When shown the radiograph establishes the diagnosis of posterior total hip replacement dislocation		
Recognises need for analgesia and urgent reduction		
States would contact anaesthetist and book patient onto emergency theatre list		
Able to describe the difference between anterior and posterior dislocation of the hip		
Able to describe the sciatic nerve is at risk during dislocation		
Able to describe that sciatic nerve injury can cause sensory loss in the leg and foot drop		
Able to describe the main branches of the sciatic nerve as tibial and common peroneal nerve		
Understands that recurrent total hip replacement dislocations may be an indication for revision total hip replacement		
Summarises the situation to the examiner		
Examiner's Global Mark	/5	
Actor's Global Mark	/5	
Total Station Mark	/30	

Learning Points

- Postoperative total hip replacement dislocation can cause compression of neurovascular structures. Careful examination of the limb is important to rule out a posterior or anterior dislocation as well as look for a neurological deficit.

- The sciatic nerve exits the greater sciatic foramen and runs between the femoral neck and the piriformis making it vulnerable during posterior dislocation. It is important to recognise sciatic nerve compression so revise the distribution of innervation of the sciatic nerve and its branches.

- It is important to find out the cause of the fall. An initial ABC approach will avoid missing life threatening problems and always look for any evidence of a head injury as it is easily missed. The patient population is normally elderly and they have multiple co-morbidities.

4.6 EMERGENCY CASES: Ward – Infection

Candidate's instructions:

A 39-year-old patient has been brought up to the ward from the emergency department with a 5-day history of left index finger pain. The finger is now red and swollen. For the last 48 hours she has felt feverish and unwell. She is a type 1 diabetic.

You are the orthopaedic foundation year doctor on called and have been asked by your registrar on call to review this patient and discuss with them.
Your brief assessment can include a short focused history, examination for important signs of infection in the finger along with data interpretation.

There will be some questions from the examiner following this.

When you attend the ward the nurse reports the following observations:-

Observations:-
HR 120   BP 95/65   RR 22   Sats 90% on 2l

Examiner's instructions:

A 39-year-old patient has been brought up to the ward from the emergency department with a 5-day history of left index finger pain. The finger is now red and swollen. For the last 48 hours she has felt feverish and unwell. She is a type 1 diabetic.

The candidate is an orthopaedic foundation year doctor on called and they have been asked by you, the registrar on-call to review this patient and report back to you.

You should allow the candidate 6 minute for assessment and then a further 2 minutes to present their findings and management plan and answer your questions.

You should ask the following questions;

1. What is the underlying pathology of flexor sheath infection?
2. What are the cardinal signs of flexor sheath infection?
3. Describe 3 risk factors of flexor sheath infection?
4. What are the complications associated with flexor sheath infection?

Actor's instructions

You are a 39-year-old patient has been brought up to the ward from the emergency department with a 5-day history of left index finger pain. Your finger is now red and swollen. For the last 48 hours you have felt feverish and unwell. You are a type 1 diabetic. Non-smoker and take no regular medications.

The candidate will ask some basic questions then proceed to examine your hand. Due to the nature of the condition the examiners will feedback the positive findings to the candidate.

4.6 EMERGENCY CASES: Ward – Infection

Task:	Achieved	Not Achieved
Describes ABC approach to patient assessment		
Establishes the background injury and whether there were any previous episodes		
Elicits the timing of onset		
Elicits the severity of pain		
Asks about systemic symptoms of fever, rigors and night sweats		
Asks about past medical history and risk factors eg; Diabetes, drug use, immunosuppression		
Offers examination of the affected hand		
States signs to observe on examination eg; finger flexed, swelling, wound, erythema		
Demonstrates assessing gross sensory function		
Demonstrates assessing gross motor function		
Demonstrates assessment of capillary refill time		
When shown the picture recognises flexor sheath infection		
Recognises need for analgesia and urgent operative washout / debridement		
Interprets observations as a sign of systemic sepsis and requests urgent antibiotics, IV fluids and urine output monitoring		
States would contact anaesthetist and book patient onto emergency theatre list		
Able to describe the pathology in flexor sheath infection		
Able to describe Kanavel's signs		
Able to describe 3 or more risk factors		
Able to describe complications of flexor sheath infection		
Summarises the situation to the examiner		
Examiner's Global Mark	/5	
Actor's Global Mark	/5	
Total Station Mark	/30	

Learning Points

- Patients with a flexor sheath infection can be very unwell and even septic. The underlying pathology is infection of the flexor sheath which, as it is a fixed space, is considered similar to a compartment syndrome.

- Kanavel's signs predict likelihood of flexor tenosynovitis as a diagnosis
    - Flexed posture of digit
    - Tenderness to palpation
    - Pain with passive extension
    - Fusiform swelling

- Examples of risk factors include diabetes, smoking, IVDU and immunosuppression

- Complications include flexion contracture/ stiffness, flexor tendon or pulley rupture, osteomyelitis

4.7 EMERGENCY CASES: Ward – Pulmonary Embolism

Candidate's instructions

A 65-year-old woman is recovering on day seven after long operative intervention for a pelvic fracture following a road traffic accident. Her post op mobility has been poor. She has developed shortness of breath and chest pain.

You are the foundation year doctor on the wards. You have been asked by the medical registrar on call to review the patient and report your findings back to them. Your brief assessment can include a short focused history, examinations for key signs and will include data interpretation.

There will be some questions from the examiner following this.

You are presented with the most recent set of observations and an ECG and CXR the nursing staff have done:

Observations:-
HR 120 BP 95/65   RR 22   Sats 90% on 2l

ECG:-   Sinus Tachycardia

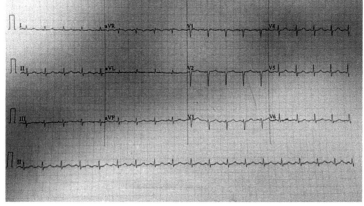

CXR

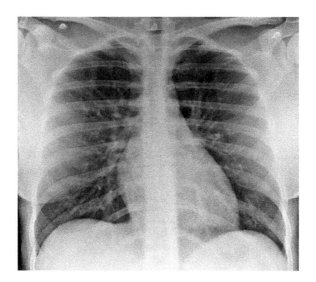

Examiner's instructions

A 65-year-old woman is recovering on day seven after operative intervention for a pelvic fracture following a road traffic accident. She has developed shortness of breath and chest pain.

The candidate is a foundation year doctor on the wards. They have been asked by the medical registrar on call to review the patient and report their findings back to them. They have been presented with the most recent set of observations and an ECG and CXR. You should allow the candidate 6 minute for assessment and then a further 2 minutes to present their findings and management plan and answer your questions.

You should ask the following questions;

1. What is are the differential diagnoses in this situation?
2. Name 3 risk factors for pulmonary embolus?
3. What radiological investigation might you request to look for pulmonary embolus?
4. What medication might be considered appropriate provided there are no contraindications?

Actor's instructions

You are a 65-year-old woman is recovering on day seven after operative intervention for a pelvic fracture following a road traffic accident. You have suddenly developed acute shortness of breath and bilateral chest pain on attempting to breathe deeply.

The candidate will ask some basic questions then proceed to examine your leg. Due to the nature of the condition the examiners will feedback the positive findings to the candidate.

4.7 EMERGENCY CASES: Ward – Pulmonary Embolism

Task:	Achieved	Not Achieved
Describes ABC approach to patient assessment		
Establishes the presenting complaint, background and operative intervention		
Elicits the timing of onset		
Asks chest pain and shortness of breath		
Elicits the severity of symptoms		
Asks about PMHx and risk factors		
Offers examination of the chest		
States signs to observe on examination eg; tachypnoea, cyanosis, accessory respiratory effort, tachycardia		
Demonstrates assessing chest examination		
Demonstrates assessing cardiac auscultation		
Demonstrates assessment distal limbs for swelling consistent with DVT		
Recognises an emergency situation and requests full set of observations		
Recognises need for oxygen and IV fluids		
Requests further investigations of bloods, ABG, ECG, CXR		
States would contact senior member of the team or Medical Registrar for urgent review		
Able to describe differentials diagnoses		
Able to describe 3 risk factors for pulmonary embolus		
Able to describe suggest CTPA for further investigation		
Able to describe use of treatment dose low molecular weight heparin provided there are no contraindications		
Summarises the situation to the examiner		
Examiner's Global Mark	/5	
Actor's Global Mark	/5	
Total Station Mark	/30	

Learning Points

- Pulmonary embolus is a high risk after orthopaedic operations especially pelvic and lower limb operations.

- An ABC approach should be taken to all acutely unwell patients and in this scenario urgent oxygen administration is required prior to contacting senior doctors.

- If pulmonary embolus is likely and in the absence of contraindications treatment dose low molecular weight heparin can be started while awaiting CTPA but should be done with the guidance of more senior doctors particularly in the context of major pelvic surgery.

4.8 EMERGENCY CASES: Ward – Neck of Femur fracture

Candidate's instructions

A 95-year-old lady has been brought up to the orthopaedic ward from the emergency department. She is normally a nursing home resident and was found by her carers on the floor. She is complaining of pain and is disorientated in time and place.

The patient has had a hip x-ray in accident and emergency. An AMTS has been done which is 6/10. The nurses have done a set of observations.

You are the foundation year doctor on call for trauma and orthopaedics and have been asked to clerk her in. Your brief assessment can include a short focused history, examinations for key signs and will include radiograph interpretation.

Observations

BP 110/70   HR 105   RR 18   Sats 90%

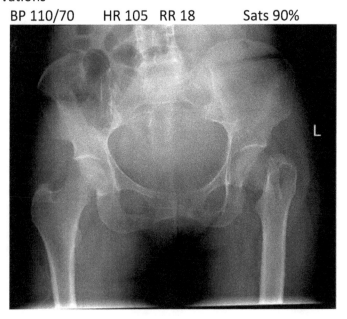

Examiner's instructions

A 95-year-old lady has been brought up to the orthopaedic ward from the emergency department. She is screaming out in pain and trying to get out of her bed. The patient has had a hip x-ray and a chest x-ray in accident and emergency. The nurses have done a set of observations.

The candidate is the foundation year doctor on call for trauma and orthopaedics and has been asked to clerk her in. They have been presented with the following x-rays and observations.

You should allow the candidate 6 minute for assessment and then a further 2 minutes to present their findings and management plan.

Actor's instructions

You are a 95-year-old lady who has been brought up to the orthopaedic ward from accident and emergency. You are normally a nursing home resident and following a fall you were found by her carers on the floor. You are in pain but disorientated in time and place and unable to fully answer any questions from the candidate.

The candidate will ask some basic questions then proceed to examine your leg. Due to the nature of the condition the examiners will feedback the positive findings to the candidate.

4.8 EMERGENCY CASES: Ward – Neck of Femur fracture

Task:	Achieved	Not Achieved
Describes ABC approach to patient assessment		
Establishes the injury and background with patient or nursing staff		
Attempts to elicit duration of time on the floor with patient or nursing staff		
Attempts to ask about non-mechanical fall symptoms such as chest pain, shortness of breath with patient or nursing staff		
Attempts to ask about past medical history and risk factors with patient or nursing staff		
Attempts to ask about pre-injury functional level		
Recognises dementia with AMTS level of 6		
Offers examination to assess for head injury and states that they would assess GCS score		
Demonstrates assessing chest examination		
Demonstrates assessing cardiac examination		
Demonstrates assessing abdominal examination		
Demonstrates assessment of pressure areas		
States that they would look for signs of fracture neck of femur including shortening and internal rotation of limb		
Demonstrates neurovascular examination of affected limb		
Requests further investigations including bloods, ECG, Pelvis and hip xrays		
Confirms fracture neck of femur on radiographs and recognises need for operative intervention on the next available trauma list		
States that they would offer analgesia, IV fluids and thromboprophylaxis and ensure patient isnil by mouth from midnight		
States would contact senior member of the team or Medical Registrar for review depending upon local policy		
Recognises the significance of a potential 'long-lie' on the floor and suggests catheterisation, urine output monitoring and U&E check		
Summarises the situation to the examiner		
Examiner's Global Mark	/5	
Actor's Global Mark	/5	
Total Station Mark	/30	

Learning Points

Patients with a fractured neck of femur present a significant workload to orthopaedic departments and the NHS. They suffer from significant comorbidities and have long inpatient stays. A more joined up approach with orthogeriatric multidisciplinary teams is now becoming the norm.

They must be carefully assessed for other medical issues that may have precipitated the fall. It is important to know the 10 point scoring system of the AMTS. Patients in this age group may have a background of dementia but always consider that a reduced AMTS could indicate a delirium and consider excluding additional problems such as head injury, urine infection or chest infection.

Management of these patients includes optimisation for early surgery, operative intervention and multidisciplinary rehabilitation.

4.9 EMERGENCY CASES: ATLS scenario

Candidate's Instructions:

A 56-year-old man has been brought by ambulance to the Emergency Department following falling from a ladder at a height of 3m.

You are the orthopaedic doctor in the trauma team and have been asked to perform a primary survey. Your brief assessment can include a short focused history, examinations for key signs and will include data interpretation.

There will be some questions from the examiner following this.

Examiner's Instructions:

A 56-year-old man has been brought by ambulance to the Emergency Department following falling from a ladder at a height of 3m.

The orthopaedic doctor in the trauma team has been asked to perform a primary survey.

If asked by the candidate for the patient's examination findings:

- Airway is clear, no abnormal sounds.

- Chest expands equally, central trachea, normal percussion note, equal normal breath sounds, no chest wall tenderness.

- Palpable radial pulse. No obvious haemorrhage sites. Soft, non-tender abdomen, no stigmata of pelvic injury. No pain in upper limbs, no pain in thighs, pain in both ankles and feet.

- Observations:-HR 120 BP 95/65   RR 22   Sats 90% on 2l

Actor's Instructions:

You are a 56-year-old man who fell from a ladder at a height of 3m whilst painting the outside of your house. You landed on both your feet onto tarmac. You were unable to get up at afterwards and your partner called for an ambulance. The ambulance crew arrived rapidly and put a cervical collar with blocks on and placed you on a stretcher and brought you to the resuscitation part of the ED.

You are aware of where you are and what happened. You can talk normally and your breathing feels normal. You have pain in both your feet and your back only. You don't have any pain in your neck, chest, abdomen or pelvis. Apart from the pain in your feet your legs feel otherwise normal. When asked if you have any pain you are very focused on the pain in your heels.

4.9 EMERGENCY CASES: ATLS scenario

Task:	Achieved	Not Achieved
Introduces self		
Checks patient's name and DOB		
Washes hands/uses alcohol gel		
Puts on gown and gloves		
Assesses airway		
Looks for obvious chest injuries		
Assesses trachea position		
Palpates chest wall bilaterally		
Percusses chest wall bilaterally		
Auscultates chest bilaterally		
Checks respiratory rate and saturations		
Assesses radial pulse		
Checks pulse and blood pressure		
Examines abdomen		
Assesses pelvis		
Examines long bones		
Assesses for external haemorrhage		
Assesses GCS		
Does not remove cervical collar and blocks		
Avoids focusing on painful feet/ sticks to ABCDE		
Examiner's Global Mark	/5	
Actor's Global Mark	/5	
Total Station Mark	/30	

Learning Points

- When performing a primary survey, you must not become distracted by other injuries (such as the likely calcaneal fractures in this scenario). These are assessed in the secondary survey, once the primary survey, and any appropriate interventions, have been undertaken

- Always consider the possibility of vertebral fractures in patients with calcaneal fractures. Given the common mechanism of a fall from height up to 10% of patients with a calcaneal fracture will have a concomitant vertebral fracture.

- The cervical spine immobilisation collar should not be removed during the primary survey unless required to undertake an intervention for the airway.

COMMUNICATION

5.1 COMMUNICATION: Consent for theatre

Candidate's Instructions:

A fit and healthy 21-year-old woman was admitted late last night with a broken ankle. She was placed in a temporary backslab and is on the trauma operating list today for "open reduction and internal fixation of the right ankle" where the fracture will be fixed with a small metal plate a series of screws.

You are the foundation year doctor in the orthopaedic team. Having seen this operation several times before your Consultant has asked you to go through the consent process with the patient. You will also need to answer any questions that patient may have.

You have 6 minutes to complete the task before being asked to summarise your consultation to the examiner.

Examiner's Instructions:

A fit and healthy 21-year-old woman was admitted late last night with a broken ankle. She was placed in a temporary backslab and is on the trauma operating list today for "open reduction and internal fixation of the right ankle" where the fracture will be fixed with a small metal plate a series of screws.

The foundation year doctor has been asked to answer the patient's questions and go through the consent process. They have seen this operation before several times and are therefore able to explain it to the patient. They need to obtain informed consent and documented proof of this by signing the consent form with the patient.

After 6 minutes stop the candidate whatever stage they are at and ask them to 'please summarize your consultation'.

Actor's Instructions:

You have fallen whilst drunk last night and been admitted the hospital with a broken right ankle. After a brief visit from the on-call consultant this morning you were informed that you are awaiting an operation to fix your broken ankle on today's trauma operating list. The consultant had to move on to the next patient and told you another doctor would return and explain it to you.

You didn't get much sleep last night as you were brought up very late from the emergency department. Your pain is under control and although you feel a bit worse for wear you are no longer drunk. You would like to know how long the operation will take and what is involved. You are alarmed by the fact that some serious risks are listed by the doctor but accept that they are part and parcel of the treatment you require once explained to you

You are currently at university and do tend to drink a bit too much and you smoke socially. You take the oral contraceptive pill but no other medications and are in general good health. You have never had an operation or anaesthetic before. This is making you very nervous about today. It doesn't help that you are tired and hungry as you were not allowed anything to eat and drink in preparation for the operation.

You have already been up on a set of crutches this morning with the physiotherapist and you found it very hard work but managed it safely.

When asked if they can put a mark on the correct leg prior to the operation you ask why that is necessary considering you have a plaster on your leg and only one of your ankle is bruised and swollen!

5.1 COMMUNICATION: Consent for theatre

Task:	Achieved	Not Achieved
Introduces him/herself		
Clarifies who they are speaking to, establishes age and occupation of the patient		
Positions themselves at appropriate distance from patient and maintains eye contact		
Explains the purpose of the consultation and what they expect to achieve		
Establishes what the patient knows so far and elicits concerns		
Clearly states the procedure and confirms with the patient the correct side and site of surgery		
Offers to mark/checks marking of surgery site		
Lists (and explains if needed) - Infection risk		
Lists (and explains if needed) - Bleeding risk		
Lists (and explains if needed) – Risk or damage to local important structures i.e. nerves, blood vessels etc.		
Lists (and explains if needed) – VTE risk		
Lists (and explains if needed) – Malunion/non-union risk		
Lists (and explains if needed) – Repeat operation risk and/removal of metalwork		
Is able to explain the options for non-surgical treatment along with the risks of not treating an unstable ankle fracture		
Uses consent form and obtains appropriate signature		
Appears professional during consultation		
Gives clear and understandable information without excessive use of jargon or acronyms		
Allows the patient to talk and ask questions without talking over them		
Ensures all patient's concerns are dealt with		
Summarises the consultation to the examiner		
Examiner's Global Mark	/5	
Actor's Global Mark	/5	
Total Station Mark	/30	

Learning Points

- Knowing the basics risks of a general orthopaedic trauma procedure are the crux of this station. Being able to explain them in simple terms to the patient rather than just listing them is what is required and what will happen in the real world.

- A knowledge of the consent process including confirming the site and nature of the operation and being able to offer advice about alternative treatment makes the candidate safe.

- Being able to obtain consent whilst stating often concerning risks (infection, repeat operation, damage to nerves) is aided by stratifying the list of risks into common (pain and swelling), less common (removal of metalwork) and rare (nerve damage).

5.2 COMMUNICATION: Counselling about thromboprophylaxis

Candidate's Instructions:

A fit and healthy 21-year-old woman was admitted 2 days ago with broken ankle she underwent surgery to fix the broken ankle (open reduction and internal fixation) yesterday and is due to be discharged home non-weight bearing in a plaster cast (below her knee).

You are the foundation year doctor in the orthopaedic team and have been asked to discharge the patient. The patient would like to know more information about preventing deep vein thrombosis (DVT) prior to going home.

You have 6 minutes to complete the task before being asked to summarise your consultation to the examiner.

Examiner's Instructions:

A fit and healthy 21-year-old woman was admitted 2 days ago with broken ankle she underwent surgery to fix the broken ankle (open reduction and internal fixation) yesterday and is due to be discharged home non-weight bearing in a plaster cast (below her knee).

The foundation year doctor has been asked to answer the patient's questions about preventing deep vein thrombosis (DVT) as part of the discharge process. The patient will voice concern about getting a DVT whilst in a plaster cast the candidate is expected to perform a Venous thrombo-embolism (VTE) assessment on the patient and explain the role of Enoxaparin injections and compression stockings.

After 6 minutes stop the candidate whatever stage they are at and ask them to 'please summarize your consultation'.

Actor's Instructions:

You have fallen whilst drunk and been admitted the hospital with a broken ankle. You underwent surgery yesterday to fix the broken bone with a combination of metal plates and screws. It was explained to you that you need to be in a plaster and cannot put any weight through that leg for the next 6 weeks. You will be walking with crutches.

You hadn't thought about Deep Vein Thrombosis (blood clot in the leg veins) until the nurse giving you your enoxaparin injection in your tummy last night explained what it was for (to reduce the risk of DVT). You have since been looking on the internet and are concerned that you are at risk. This has worried you as your parents neighbour had died two years ago after developing a blood clot (you don't know the specific circumstances of this). You also think that your aunt may have developed a blood clot after a period in hospital but seemed to recover ok. You are currently at university and do tend to drink a bit too much and you smoke socially. You take the oral contraceptive pill but no other medications and are in general good health and good physical shape (i.e. not clinically obese).

The doctor will attempt to assess your risk of developing a DVT by asking you some questions and will explain methods by which the risk can be reduced. You can help steer the consultation appropriately by asking pertinent questions such as:
- Do you think I am at risk of getting a DVT?
- What can I do to prevent it?

You are not particularly needle phobic but don't like the idea of being 'stabbed' every day and you are not keen on wearing the stocking in bed at night as they make you hot.

Finally, (if there is time) you were hoping to fly out to Spain for a holiday with friends next month and you would like to know if this is a good idea.

5.2 COMMUNICATION: Counselling about thromboprophylaxis

Task:	Achieved	Not Achieved
Introduces him/herself		
Clarifies who they are speaking to, establishes age and occupation of the patient		
Positions themselves at appropriate distance from patient and maintains eye contact		
Explains the purpose of the consultation and what they expect to achieve		
Establishes what the patient knows so far and elicits concerns		
Explains that assessing someone's VTE risk is a balanced risk of developing a DVT versus bleeding risk of treatment		
Establishes risk of being immobilized and non-weight bearing in plaster cast		
Establishes risk of medication eg; Oral contraceptive pill		
Establishes no major bleeding risks		
Asks about personal history of VTE		
Asks about family history of VTE		
Makes appropriate judgment of the patients DVT risk and gives the appropriate advice		
Explains how low molecular weight heparin works in simple terms and describes a typical dose regimen		
Explains how compression stocks work		
Suggests other methods to lower risk (hydration, staying mobile, avoiding alcohol)		
Appears professional during consultation		
Gives clear and understandable information without excessive use of jargon or acronyms		
Allows the patient to talk and ask questions without talking over them		
Ensures all patient's concerns are dealt with		
Summarises the consultation to the examiner		
Examiner's Global Mark	/5	
Actor's Global Mark	/5	
Total Station Mark	/30	

Learning Points

- Knowing the basics of a VTE risk assessment are key – you have to make your own judgment call for this particular patient balancing her risk factors against any bleeding risk.

- A basic knowledge of the action and prescription of enoxaparin and compression stockings is also important as these details are important to the patient (when do I take it? How often? When can I stop?)

- While this isn't a particularly confrontational consultation there is the need here to stand by your convictions and not change your advice when the patient doesn't necessarily like the medical advice you have given them (doesn't like needles, stocking make them too hot and would quite like to fly abroad!)

5.3 COMMUNICATION: Counselling about bisphosphonates

Candidate's Instructions:

A 78-year-old woman recently fell on an outstretched hand and suffered from a distal radius fracture. She was seen in fracture clinic where they opted for conservative management. Given that the fracture occurred without significant trauma, the orthopaedic team have advised that she starts on a bisphosphonate. They have advised her to see her GP to start the medication.

You are the foundation year doctor working in general practice. Please discuss the medication with the patient and address any concerns.

You have 6 minutes to complete the task before being asked to summarise your consultation to the examiner.

Examiner's Instructions:

A 78-year-old woman with a recent history of fragility fracture has been asked to attend her GP to start a bisphosphonate. She has done some reading online about bisphosphonates and is very concerned about starting on the medication. She will be particularly concerned about the risk of osteonecrosis of the jaw and atypical femoral fractures.

The candidate should be aware that the risk of osteoporotic fragility fracture far outweighs the risk of atypical fragility fractures and osteonecrosis of the jaw in this instance.

The candidate should give adequate advice on how the medication should be taken. Alendronic acid is the first line biologic in the UK. It is given as a once weekly preparation. The BNF advises "Tablets should be swallowed whole with plenty of water while sitting or standing; to be taken on an empty stomach at least 30 minutes before breakfast (or another oral medicine); patient should stand or sit upright for at least 30 minutes after taking tablet"

After 6 minutes stop the candidate whatever stage they are at and ask them to 'please summarize your consultation'.

Actor's Instructions:

You are a 78-year-old woman who recently had an innocuous fall at home onto your left hand. Unfortunately, you fractured your wrist and it has been put in a cast. The orthopaedic team were happy with the alignment of the fracture but were concerned that it didn't take much force to break the bone. They suggested that you see your GP to start a type of medication called a bisphosphonate.

In fracture clinic they didn't explain anything about these medications but you have done your own research online and are quite concerned about the potential side effects. You have read that they can "rot your jaw" and even can cause unusual hip fractures in some cases. You are baffled why anyone would think these medications are a good idea as it sounds like they do more harm than good. You just need to be more careful at home and avoid falling.

Initially you will be quite adamant that you don't want to start the medication but with proper explanation of the risks and a sympathetic ear you will be willing to try it. A friend of yours has osteoporosis and is given a medication that they take by injection once every 6 months called denosumab. Can't you have that instead?

5.3 COMMUNICATION: Counselling about bisphosphonates

Task:	Achieved	Not Achieved
Introduces him/herself		
Clarifies who they are speaking to, establishes age and occupation of the patient		
Positions themselves at appropriate distance from patient and maintains eye contact		
Explains the purpose of the consultation and what they expect to achieve		
Establishes what the patient knows so far and elicits concerns		
Allows the patient time to talk without interruption		
Recommends that the patient start an oral bisphosphonate (alendronate would be first line)		
Explains that the medication is only taken once per week		
Advises that the medication is taken on an empty stomach at least 30 minutes before breakfast		
Advises the patient to drink plenty of water alongside when taking their bisphosphonate		
Advises that the patient should remain upright for 30 minutes after taking the medication		
Reassures the patient appropriately that the risk of osteonecrosis of the jaw is extremely low		
Addresses the patient's concerns about atypical femoral fractures appropriately		
Advises that the patient should take oral supplementation of calcium and vitamin D alongside the bisphosphonate		
Addresses patient's questions about denosumab appropriately		
Appears professional during consultation		
Gives clear and understandable information without excessive use of jargon or acronyms		
Allows the patient to talk and ask questions without talking over them		
Ensures all patient's concerns are dealt with		
Summarises the consultation to the examiner		
Examiner's Global Mark	/5	
Actor's Global Mark	/5	
Total Station Mark	/30	

Learning Points

- Atypical femoral fractures have been seen in patients with prolonged bisphosphonate use but the risk is low. The risk of osteoporotic fragility fracture in a patient like this far outweighs the risk of atypical femoral fracture and treatment should therefore be given. The MHRA advice states "The risk of osteonecrosis of the jaw is substantially greater for patients receiving intravenous bisphosphonates in the treatment of cancer than for patients receiving oral bisphosphonates for osteoporosis or Paget's disease".

- Current NICE guidelines on secondary prevention of osteoporotic fractures [TA161] do not require a DEXA scan to be performed before commencing a bisphosphonate in women over the age of 75 who have suffered a fragility fracture.

- Denosumab is licensed for the treatment of osteoporosis in the UK but current NICE guidelines only recommend its use in patients who have a contra-indication or intolerance to oral bisphosphonates which are still the first line treatment for osteoporosis.

5.4 COMMUNICATION: Counselling about fragility fracture and DEXA scan

Candidate's Instructions:

A 74-year-old woman was referred to the metabolic bone clinic for investigation of osteoporosis having sustained a vertebral wedge fracture at L2 without trauma. Scans at the time excluded malignancy as a possible cause of the fracture. She has been seen once in the clinic but was sent for a DEXA scan. The results are shown below.

She has returned today to get the results. Please explain the results of the scan to her and discuss possible treatment options. You are not expected to take a full medical history but may wish to ask about other risk factors for osteoporosis.

	T-Score	Z-Score
Hip	-2.8	-1.2
Lumbar Spine	-1.6	-0.3

You have 6 minutes to complete the task before being asked to summarise your consultation to the examiner.

5.4 COMMUNICATION: Counselling about fragility fracture and DEXA scan

Examiner's Instructions:

A 74-year-old woman with a recent L2 wedge fracture has recently had a DEXA scan. The results are shown below and confirm osteoporosis according to WHO criteria.

The reading at the spine shows osteopaenia but caution should be used in interpreting this as the vertebral fracture can lead to a falsely elevated reading in this region. The L2 vertebra should be excluded from the analysis of the lumbar spine bone mineral density.

The patient has several risk factors for osteoporosis including her age, sex, past use of glucocorticoids and current use of carbamazepine. This patient should be started on secondary prevention therapy with a bisphosphonate. Oral alendronic acid would be first line according to current NICE guidelines.

After 6 minutes stop the candidate whatever stage they are at and ask them to 'please summarize your consultation'.
5.4 COMMUNICATION: Counselling about fragility fracture and DEXA scan

Actor's Instructions:

You are a 74-year-old woman who recently had a vertebral fracture at L2. The fracture happened about two months ago and the pain is much better now. You are quite concerned that it might happen again. You have had a DEXA scan and want to know the results. You want to know if you have osteoporosis.

You have a past medical history includes
1. trigeminal neuralgia treated with carbamazepine
2. Polymyalgia rheumatica – which was treated with steroids for two years but you are now off treatment
3. Osteoarthritis – for which you take occasional neurofen over the counter

You never smoked and don't drink regular alcohol. You do not have a family history of osteoporosis.

You want to know if any of the medications you have been taking could have be contributing to the osteoporosis. You enjoy regular walking in your local park and are concerned that you will have to stop this because of the osteoporosis. You sometimes get pain in your hands and wonder if that is due to osteoporosis too.

5.4 COMMUNICATION: Counselling about fragility fracture and DEXA scan

Task:	Achieved	Not Achieved
Introduces him/herself		
Clarifies who they are speaking to, establishes age and occupation of the patient		
Positions themselves at appropriate distance from patient and maintains eye contact		
Explains the purpose of the consultation and what they expect to achieve		
Establishes what the patient knows so far and elicits concerns		
Explains the results of the DEXA scan appropriately		
Explains what osteoporosis is		
Asks the patient about their past medical history		
Asks about previous fragility fractures specifically		
Takes a focused drug history		
Takes a social history of smoking and alcohol use		
Correctly identifies the drugs that may be contributing to the osteoporosis (prednisolone and carbamazepine)		
Recommends treatments including bisphosphonates		
Elicits patient's concerns about activity levels		
Re-assures patient appropriately that she should continue her regular walking and that load bearing exercise can improve bone mineral density		
Appears professional during consultation		
Gives clear and understandable information without excessive use of jargon or acronyms		
Allows the patient to talk and ask questions without talking over them		
Ensures all patient's concerns are dealt with		
Summarises the consultation to the examiner		
Examiner's Global Mark	/5	
Actor's Global Mark	/5	
Total Station Mark	/30	

Learning Points

- When interpreting a DEXA scan the T-Score compares the bone mineral density to a cohort of healthy 30-year-old women whereas the Z-Score compares to an age and sex matched population.

- The World Health Organisation classifies T-scores of greater than -1 as normal; between -1 and -2.5 as osteopaenia and less than -2.5 as osteoporosis

- Other common risk factors for osteoporosis include low BMI, previous fracture, history of hip fracture in either parent, smoking, glucocorticoid use, rheumatoid arthritis and consumption of more than 3 units of alcohol per day.

5.5 COMMUNICATION: Counselling - new diagnosis of rheumatoid arthritis

Candidate's Instructions:

A 30-year-old woman was referred to the rheumatology clinic with an 8-week history of joint pain and swelling affecting the hands, wrists and knees bilaterally. The history and examination was suggestive of inflammatory arthritis and she was sent for further investigations. Blood tests showed a strongly positive anti-CCP antibody and ultrasound confirmed active synovitis at the wrists and MCP joints bilaterally. She has returned to clinic today to get the results and discuss the next steps.

You are the foundation year doctor in clinic and have been asked to explain the diagnosis and discuss the next steps with the patient.

You have 6 minutes to complete the task before being asked to summarise your consultation to the examiner.

5.5 COMMUNICATION: Counselling - new diagnosis of rheumatoid arthritis

Examiner's Instructions:

A 30-year-old woman with an 8-week history of joint pain and swelling in a distribution that is typical for rheumatoid arthritis (RA) has attended clinic today. She has been seen once before and investigations were requested. These have confirmed a diagnosis of RA. She has returned to clinic today to get the results and discuss the treatment options.

The candidate should explain the diagnosis in simple terms minimising the use of jargon or where medical terms are used give a lay explanation for them.

The candidate should be aware that modern treatment strategies advocate starting treatment with disease modifying anti-rheumatic drugs (DMARDs) early to prevent permanent damage. The most commonly used first line drug is methotrexate and this should at least be discussed. However, methotrexate is potentially teratogenic and the candidate should explain that alternatives are available without having to give specific examples.

The candidate should appropriately re-assure the patient that the risk of her future children being affected by the disease is low.

After 6 minutes stop the candidate whatever stage they are at and ask them to 'please summarize your consultation'.
5.5 COMMUNICATION: Counselling - new diagnosis of rheumatoid arthritis

Actor's Instructions:

You are a 30-year-old woman and have been experiencing joint pain and swelling that has developed gradually over the past 8 weeks. It has been affecting your hands, wrists and knees bilaterally. You saw a different doctor in clinic two weeks ago who arranged some investigations including blood tests and an ultrasound scan. One of the things that the previous doctor mentioned they were considering was rheumatoid arthritis.

You don't know a great deal about rheumatoid arthritis but would like to know more. You would like to know about the condition and if anything you have done might have caused it to develop (if asked, you are a non-smoker).

You think that your grandmother had rheumatoid arthritis and she was very disabled by the condition. In particular, her hands were quite deformed. You are worried that this might happen to you.

You would like to know what treatments are available for the condition and if there will be any side effects from the treatment. You hope to start a family one day and are concerned that you will pass the disease onto your children. You currently work in an office and are concerned about the impact of the disease on your job. You also are a keen cyclist and wonder if you should give up cycling.

5.5 COMMUNICATION: Counselling - new diagnosis of rheumatoid ar

Task:	Achieved	Not Achieved
Introduces him/herself		
Clarifies who they are speaking to, establishes age and occupation of the patient		
Positions themselves at appropriate distance from patient and maintains eye contact		
Explains the purpose of the consultation and what they expect to achieve		
Establishes what the patient knows so far		
Explains the diagnosis of rheumatoid arthritis. Avoids the use of jargon – if technical terms are used they must also be explained in lay terms		
Reassures the patient that nothing they have done has caused them to develop arthritis		
Elicits concern that the patient will end up like her grandmother.		
Re-assures the patient that with modern treatment outcomes are much improved and she is very unlikely to be as severely affected by the disease as her grandmother		
Explains briefly how rheumatoid arthritis is treated (must mention either methotrexate or DMARDs)		
Discusses a multidisciplinary approach to the treatment of RA (involving pharmacist, physiotherapist, podiatrist etc.)		
Lists some of the side effects of methotrexate or other DMARDs (nausea, hair thinning, liver toxicity, increased risk of infections, need for blood test monitoring) – must mention at least two to score the mark		
Identifies that methotrexate is teratogenic and explains that a different treatment should be used instead		
Re-assures the patient appropriately about her risk of her children developing the condition		
Elicits concern that the patient will have to give up cycling and reassures the patient about the benefits of exercise in RA		
Appears professional during consultation		

Gives clear and understandable information without excessive use of jargon or acronyms		
Allows the patient to talk and ask questions without talking over them		
Ensures all patient's concerns are dealt with		
Summarises the consultation to the examiner		
Examiner's Global Mark	/5	
Actor's Global Mark	/5	
Total Station Mark	/30	

Learning Points

- Rheumatoid arthritis commonly presents as a symmetrical polyarthritis affecting predominantly the small joints

- Early treatment with disease modifying anti-rheumatic drugs is associated with better clinical outcomes and as such contemporary treatment algorithms advocate prompt referral to a specialist and early initiation of DMARDs.

- Rheumatoid arthritis affects approximately 1% of the population. If you have a first degree relative with the condition your risk of developing RA is increased by approximately 3-5 times. However, this means you are still much more likely to never get the condition than you are to develop it.

CPSIA information can be obtained
at www.ICGtesting.com
Printed in the USA
LVHW052324301118
598801LV00010B/424/P